THREE LITTLE
COWBOYS

THE JOURNEY OF A YOUNG MOM
THROUGH HER BATTLE WITH CANCER

THREE LITTLE
COWBOYS

ALLYSON HENDRICKSON

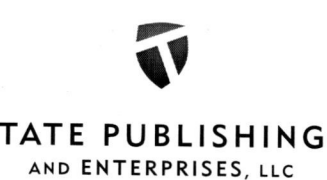

TATE PUBLISHING
AND ENTERPRISES, LLC

The Three Little Cowboys
Copyright © 2015 by Allyson Hendrickson. All rights reserved.

No part of this publication may be reproduced, stored in a retrieval system or transmitted in any way by any means, electronic, mechanical, photocopy, recording or otherwise without the prior permission of the author except as provided by USA copyright law.

This book is designed to provide accurate and authoritative information with regard to the subject matter covered. This information is given with the understanding that neither the author nor Tate Publishing, LLC is engaged in rendering legal, professional advice. Since the details of your situation are fact dependent, you should additionally seek the services of a competent professional.

The opinions expressed by the author are not necessarily those of Tate Publishing, LLC.

Published by Tate Publishing & Enterprises, LLC
127 E. Trade Center Terrace | Mustang, Oklahoma 73064 USA
1.888.361.9473 | www.tatepublishing.com

Tate Publishing is committed to excellence in the publishing industry. The company reflects the philosophy established by the founders, based on Psalm 68:11,
 "The Lord gave the word and great was the company of those who published it."

Book design copyright © 2015 by Tate Publishing, LLC. All rights reserved.
Cover design by Roland Caballero
Interior design by Mary Jean Archival

Published in the United States of America

ISBN: 978-1-68142-221-3
Biography & Autobiography / Personal Memoirs
15.05.08

Thursday, March 22, 2007

So...I GAVE UP AND GOT a blog. Everybody's doing it, right?!?!?

I am 31 years old. I love Jesus and my church. I love my husband and my kids. I love Texas, dessert, bedtime, good books, a clean house, and the occasional margarita. We live within driving distance of our family, but not too close, so a blog seems like a good way for people we love to keep up with the craziness that is our life! 3 little boys call me "Mommy." They are the sunshine in my life for sure! For blogging purposes, I will reference them by their nicknames: Goliath (5 yrs. old), Little Middle (2 yrs. old), and Baby (16 months). Unless you know us, you are probably wondering "Why 'Goliath'?" Our oldest son weighed 8 lbs, 12 oz. at birth and has consistently grown into a preschool linebacker. He is husky and strong—a gentle giant—and we hope he grows up to play for the NFL so he can take care of us when we're old.

Life with 3 preschoolers is fun and crazy and exhausting. We laugh a lot, cry a little, and my story is worth telling (doesn't every parent think that?). Case in point: Although I try to avoid taking all 3 boys to the grocery store if at all possible, the other day we were out of chicken and pickle chips. We can not live without either, so we made a grocery run. At the checkout counter, I got the usual comment from the cashier: "3 boys, huh? You sure do have your hands full!" To which Goliath replied: "And this isn't all, either. We have a dog, and a daddy, too!"

Until next time…

Happy Easter

Sunday, April 08, 2007

WHEN I SURVEY THE WONDROUS cross On which the Prince of glory died My richest gain I count but loss and pour contempt on all my pride.

See, from His head, His hands, His feet Sorrow and love flow mingled down. Did e'er such love and sorrow meet Or thorns compose so rich a crown?

Were the whole realm of nature mine, That were a present far too small. Love, so amazing, so divine, Demands my soul, my life, my all.

Happy Easter!

On My Heart

Thursday, May 03, 2007

Just a few Scriptures that have been on my heart lately…

> Teach me your way, O Lord, and I will walk in your truth; give me an undivided heart, that I may fear your name. I will praise you, O Lord my God, with all my heart; I will glorify your name forever. For great is your love toward me. (Psalm 86:11–13)

> Because of the Lord's great love we are not consumed, for his compassions never fail. They are new every morning; great is your faithfulness. (Lamentations 3:22–23)

> See, I have engraved you on the palms of my hands. (Isaiah 49:16)

> Find rest, O my soul, in God alone; my hope comes from him. He alone is my rock and my salvation. He is my fortress, I will not be shaken. (Psalm 62:5–6)

Long Time No Blog

Saturday, July 21, 2007

You may have noticed it's been a while since my last post. You may even be wondering what's up? Here, in compact form, is an update on the last 3 weeks: 3 weeks ago, Hubby was out of town on business. I woke up, started my day like normal, and felt a shooting pain in my back. It started at my shoulder blade and went all the way down to my waist. In true form, I took 2 Motrin. The pain intensified and started moving around through my rib cage and up toward my heart. I went online and googled "heart attack symptoms." The pain got worse. I called Hubby in tears. He called a friend from church, who showed up at my house within 15 minutes, loaded me and the boys up, and drove us to the hospital. Long story short, at the end of a 14-hour stay in the ER, the doctors couldn't say what had caused the excruciating pain. They DID say that the scans they had ordered had revealed a ping-pong ball size mass on my left ovary. They wrote a prescription for a painkiller and sent me home with instructions to call my ob-gyn.

The following week I saw my dr. She read over the report, looked at the pictures, and said, "Honey, that's no ping-pong ball. That's a peach." She ordered blood tests to check for "tumor markers" (a frightening term that indicates elevated levels of certain proteins where tumors may be present), and promised to call me with the results.

I waited four days. When she called, she reported that the test results were fairly normal. I breathed a sigh of relief. Then, she went on to say that she would be consulting with a gynecologist-oncologist to get his opinion on whether or not surgery would be necessary. She is familiar with me and the pace at which my life requires me to run, and agreed that if surgery could at all be avoided, we would not do it.

Less than 24 hours later, surgery was being scheduled. The oncologist apparently was of the opinion that something that has grown from nothing to peach-size in less than a year (since my last check-up) should be removed asap. He also advised against further testing or doing a biopsy pre-surgery, on the chance that a needle would puncture the growth and possibly leak cancer cells. Yup. Let's not go there.

That brings me to today. Surgery will be on August 7, and suddenly it seems like every detail of my life points to that date and the recommended six (!!!) weeks of recovery time that follows. Plans are being made for my mother to come and stay. I have had to call my boss and say I may not be there for the beginning of school. I am overwhelmed at the thought of all that needs to be done before then: school shopping, house cleaning, lots of meals in the freezer. I do not know what the future holds. I do not understand why God allows what He does. I do not have a real grasp on what this means for me or my family. Here's what I do know: I serve a God who loves me and is as unsurprised by this as I am taken aback. My God had each and every day of my life mapped out long before I was born. He knows the number of hairs on my head, each thought that I think, and He promises to be with me no matter what. He has a plan, a purpose, for what I am going through, and He only waits to see what I will do with my circumstances. Will I wonder and doubt and question His sovereignty, or will I trust His plan and rest in His arms?

> I will lift up my eyes to the hills—where does my help come from? My help comes from the Lord, the Maker of heaven and earth. (Psalm 121:1–2) http://www.youtube.com/watch?v=FtAjrNqEsoM

Diagnosis

Wednesday, August 15, 2007

August 7 has come and gone, and I am resting at home. When the doctor said I would need to take it easy for a while, she wasn't kidding! I am 8 days out, and still unable to drive a car, load the washing machine, or pick up Baby. Each day is a little bit easier, and full recovery is in sight. Or was. After I had surgery last Tuesday, the doctor made her rounds to my room on Thursday morning. My mom was with me at the time (she and Hubby were taking turns sitting with me and staying with the kids), and we heard only 6 words: "I have bad news. It's cancer." It was like watching a movie in slow motion—I remember thinking that surely the lab had mixed up results (similar to how the nurse had mixed up room numbers the day before and had tried to deliver a newborn baby to me for nursing!!!). Now, nearly a week later, I still feel like that: this MUST be someone else's life. I saw a gynecologic oncologist this morning. He is listed on D Magazine's top gyn-onc list and comes highly recommended by my own doctor. We liked him fine, but he sure wasn't the down-home, how're-the-kids-doing, come-by-and-say-hi type we are used to! He had received and reviewed the final pathology report from last week's surgery. In discussing my "case," which by the way, seems to be very interesting to the local medical community, he admitted that it's not at all black and white. The cancer seems to be "middle of the road"—not the worst type, not the best. The pathology showed the tumor had spread to my bladder, but they don't know how aggressive or to what degree. The only way to find that out is through another surgery, which will take place 2 weeks from now (just DAYS after Goliath starts kindergarten). After the operation he will know exactly what is going on and how best to treat it. If there was ever a time I could identify with Job, it is now! I absolutely can not wrap my mind around what God could possibly be thinking in allowing me to have cancer. I am comforted in knowing that "Just as the heavens are higher than the earth, so are my ways higher than your ways and my thoughts higher than your thoughts" (Isaiah 55:9). It is so hard not to worry, though—especially about the precious boys God gave me to raise. What I want most in these next few weeks is normalcy. The ability to run my household, play with my kids, and do all the other things that make my life what it is. I do NOT—WILL NOT—want to be defined by this sickness or let it change the kind of wife or mother I desire to be. As I travel farther down this road, I will do my best to keep up with blogging with the hopes that my journey will be helpful to someone else. In the meantime, thanks for reading and for praying.

No Mistakes

Thursday, August 16, 2007

I wish I could say I wrote this, but I didn't. My grandmother—a great lady and one of my best friends—sent this to me via e-mail. It spells out my heart and is worth sharing.

> My Father's way may twist and turn, My heart may throb and ache,
> But in my soul I'm glad I know, He maketh no mistake.
>
> My cherished plans may go astray, My hopes may fade away,
> But still I'll trust my Lord to lead
> For He doth know the way.
>
> Though night be dark and it may seem
> That day will never break;
> I'll pin my faith, my all in Him,
> He maketh no mistake.
>
> There is so much now I cannot see
> My eyesight is far too dim;

Three Little Cowboys

But come what may, I'll simply trust
And leave it all to Him.

For by and by the mist will lift and plain it all He'll make
Through all the way, though dark to me, He made not one mistake.

Job

Monday, August 20, 2007

Hubby and I were reading the Bible last night, sort of randomly (do you ever do that? Just flip through and wait for God to throw something at you?). In my flipping, I ended up in the book of Job (appropriate, huh?). Job 33 tells of Job's friend Elihu offering "advice." Some friend. What struck me was not so much the verses I read, but the commentary about them in my trusty NIV Life Application Study Bible. It says this:

"Being informed brings a sense of security. It's natural to want to know what's happening in our lives. Job wanted to know what was going on, why he was suffering. In previous chapters, we sense his frustration. Elihu claimed to have the answer for Job's biggest question, "Why doesn't God tell me what is happening?" Elihu told Job that God was trying to answer him, but he was not listening. Elihu misjudged God on this point. If God were to answer all our questions, we would not be adequately tested. What if God had said, "Job, Satan's going to test you and afflict you, but in the end you'll be healed and get everything back?" Job's greatest test was not the pain, but that he did not know WHY he was suffering. Our greatest test may be that we must trust God's goodness even though we don't understand why our lives are going a certain way. We must learn to trust in GOD who is good and not in the goodness of life." I want to trust the goodness of God, and know that at the end of the day, He is still sovereign. I want to rest peacefully, assured that He is taking care of things even if it doesn't seem that way. I want to have huge faith and live this life in such a way that I only point to Him. Surgery 2 will be on August 30. Please pray that the next few days will be time well spent with those I love most!

Something to Be Thankful For

Thursday, August 23, 2007

I WAS GOING TO POST about the events of yesterday, which included telling my children that their Mommy has cancer. But TODAY…I have something to be thankful for and it seems much more cheerful to share that instead. So… Goliath starts kindergarten on Monday. No child in the history of the world has been better prepared for kindergarten: we've talked about it until he probably wants to skip it entirely. We draw pictures (hanging on the kitchen wall), we play at the school playground, and we even wrote a song. The time is finally here!!! I have prayed for Goliath's kindergarten teacher for a while, asking God to send the perfect person to meet his needs and make this all-important year a fantastic experience. Today, we met that person and I believe God answered prayer. We went to "Stop & Drop" at the school. The idea is to drop off your school supplies and stop to meet your teacher. His classroom is PERFECT for him—everything I imagined it would be. His whole face lit up to see his name on the bulletin board, labeling his locker (which I didn't have until the 5th grade), and identifying his very own desk! He loved the blocks, the books, the helper chart, and even the big tree in the corner. Ms. L talked to him exactly at his level, made him feel welcome, and we left there "just a little scared but lots of excited" about our new adventure. This mama is so grateful to serve a God who cares about kindergarten!

What Tomorrow Holds

Wednesday, August 29, 2007

You've heard the old saying, "I don't know what tomorrow holds, but I know who holds tomorrow"? Truth is, I don't know what tomorrow holds. It is Surgery 2 day. It will be long and filled with unknowns. It will be a sterile operating room and a small waiting room filled with anxious loved ones. It will be friends and family waiting for news and it will be me, asking for a miracle. Where will God be tomorrow? He will be in every aspect of my day. He will be with my medical team and in the surgeon's hands. He will sit with my husband and our parents in the waiting room. He will go with me into surgery, and cover me with love and grace no matter what the outcome.

> Be strong and courageous. Do not be terrified, do not be discouraged, for the Lord your God will be with you wherever you go. (Joshua 1:9)
>
> So do not fear, for I am with you; do not be dismayed, for I am your God. I will strengthen you and help you; I will uphold you with my righteous right hand. (Isaiah 41:10)

I love this song—"Uncreated One" by Chris Tomlin (so sorry that I don't know how to post a video except to link to it). The refrain is my prayer for tomorrow and the days that follow: O Great God, be glorified Our lives laid down Yours magnified O Great God, be lifted high There is none like you. http://www.youtube.com/watch?v=PE_yTzv4-RU One more thing before tomorrow: THANK YOU. You know who you are. You have prepared meals and fed my family. You have been to the grocery store for diapers and dog food. You've brought books and magazines to help pass the long hours in bed. You have made phone calls and sent e-mails and written cards. And most of all, you have prayed. Words are inadequate to describe the great outpouring of love we have experienced these last few weeks. Our church family, our friends, our family, and people we don't even know...thank you for ministering to us. We continue to ask for your prayers and anticipate a time that we witness God's answer!

Update from the family

Friday, August 31, 2007

While we are scared to be messing with the blog, my wife's outlet for all purposes, I felt it necessary as I want the world to know what God has done.

The surgery was a great success. The doctor informed us that he was unable to locate any further Cancer, and that there was no evidence of any spreading. This is I believe a great miracle from God, and I can do nothing but praise him for this. He did multiple biopsies and we will not have the results until the end of next week, but until then, my faith is strong that we will once again have the response we have asked God for.

How can we ever thank so many who have prayed and provided for us? The Prayers, gifts, calls, and unbelievable outpouring of love have humbled us and blessed us beyond anything I would have ever imagined. I have never witnessed the spirit of God move so much in my own life, there is evidence of it in my every footstep. I thank God for my wonderful wife, and I thank him for the wonderful friends and family that are so faithful to us. I wrote a poem that I would like to add to this post for everyone to read. I just want the world to know how awesome my wife is, how proud of her I am, and how much I thank God each day for her!

Thank you all once more… hubby…

There is a Tree in my life
when I found her she was the answer to my prayers
the fruit I had tasted had left me empty, lacking in so many ways
but the fruit she provided replenished me, it healed my wounds
falling down, lacking in faith she is always there for me to lean against
she has fruit and strength for more than me,
ever faithful, ever enduring
ever loving she strengthens us all
when I waver, when confusion surrounds me
she is there standing firm and her branches point the way
there is nothing my tree cannot do,
multitudes seek out her wisdom
only I can see what I wish to say
how much she means, how amazing she is
who can ever be like her? she is the tree of the ages, blessed by God as she blesses
others with her resolve, with her ever enduring faith
she carries the thorn for us all
yet she stands firm, and my tears provide the nourishment she now needs
Love is when another's happiness is essential to your own
and I am broken

Home

Monday, September 03, 2007

JUST A QUICK UPDATE… I am home. The doctor released me this morning, and I spent most of the day resting in my own bed while my mom and my brother took the boys to the zoo. When they got home, they seemed just as glad to see me as I was to see them. I am in "recovery mode" now. I am tired, physically and emotionally. I am glad to be back where I belong, where the healing process will be somewhat easier. Thank you again for your prayers—they matter. I will update more in the next few days…

Staples, Blood Clots, and an Office Visit

Saturday, September 08, 2007

Well, I've put off blogging as long as I can. After yesterday, I feel like I have something to write about beside pain meds and restless nights. Yesterday, I had an appointment in the oncologist's office to have the staples removed from my incision. My mom and I dropped off the 2 younger boys at their first day of preschool (another post for another time) and headed into Dallas. The office is just behind the hospital where I had surgery, so we knew where we were going and were blessed with good traffic, and arrived 20 minutes early. We ended up waiting over an hour. Don't you HATE that?!? Apparently, the staple-removal case before me was rendered immobile after surgery and getting her set up took quite a while. Unfortunately, all that waiting gave me plenty of time to watch the people coming into the office. Now, obviously—it you're there at all, you're in a bad place. Duh. But the women I saw…well, here's a sample conversation that I overheard:

Lady 1 (already waiting but spotting a friend): Mary Alice, how ARE you?!?!?

Lady 2 (just arrived and signing in): Well, Wanda, I'll tell you. I'm not that great today. I don't have any PLATELETS.

Lady 1: What?!? What happened?

Lady 2: I've switched chemo meds again. And the new drug has messed up my blood, and I've had to have 3 units of blood. Each unit takes 2 hours to give, plus another hour-and-a-half between units for testing and typing. I'm in here today for more testing and I'm so worried that I'll have to go back to the hospital.

Lady 1: Tsk, tsk. What happened with the D-drug?

Lady 2: Oh, the D-drug was just terrible. I couldn't get out of bed for days. I had no energy. I just couldn't do ANYTHING.

Lady 1: You know he (the doctor) isn't here today.

Lady 2: Yes, I know he's still on vacation. I heard he's having a fabulous time. I'll tell you, after each blood unit, I would stop by Krispy Kreme on the way home. I would buy a dozen donuts and eat every single one!

Lady 1: ha ha ha

Lady 2: Harold would say, "Honey, are you hungry?" And I would tell him, "No, not really." Then we would drive through Krispy Kreme anyway. They were delicious. Both ladies laugh like this is the funniest thing they have ever heard. I'm certain that they are both wearing wigs. I am depressed. When the sad surgery case finally was done, it was my turn. I don't mind saying that I was pretty worked up about having staples removed. The doctor had told me in the hospital that it wouldn't hurt a bit, but I was not buying it. While the nurse was prepping to take the staples out, my mom mentioned to her that I had been experiencing leg pain. Well. That one sentence threw the entire office into a tizzy. Marilyn and Vicki and Jerri Ann went nuts. Other assorted nurses and assistants were rushing in and out of the room, looking worried. One of them pushed on my feet. "Does this hurt? Does this hurt? Does this hurt?" I wanted to punch her in the nose.

Three Little Cowboys

Someone finally explained that they were concerned about blood clots, a common and serious occurrence after surgery. They paged the doctor, who ordered a doppler scan for my legs that had to be done TODAY. Nobody cared that I had 3 children who needed to be picked up from school in a timely fashion. They removed the staples and sent us on our merry way back to the hospital. I had to be re-admitted to the hospital as an outpatient case. When the clerk asked if I had been to Medical City before, I almost laughed. Been here? I just left here! This whole time, Mom was making frantic phone calls to Hubby to try to make a plan for retrieving the children. There was more paperwork, and we were sent upstairs. No waiting. I couldn't believe it. It is so irritating to me that the medical community seems to have no real sense of timeliness! But that precious sono tech let us right in, and we were done in less than 30 minutes. The rules are that a physician has to review each scan and sign off on it before the patient is allowed to leave. I think the tech felt sorry for me, because she said, "I'm no rookie, and I can't see anything here to worry about. Ya'll go ahead and go, and if I'm wrong, we'll call you." Hubs had to get the little boys from preschool, but Mom and I made it to the elementary school to get Goliath, with a few moments to spare for Chipotle chips and guac in the car. Still no explanation on the leg pain, though. Oh—in the middle of the frantic office visit, I did ask about the pathology reports. No sign of them yet, so we are resigned to more waiting. I'm good at some things—like making up preschool songs, baking goodies, and loving my family. But I stink at being a cancer patient. All this laying around and not doing anything useful is really getting under my skin. I do realize how important resting is, and I'm doing my best... really. I miss my life, and if you're in my life, I miss you.

It Takes a Village

Friday, September 14, 2007

IT IS QUIET THIS MORNING. Hubby is at work, and all 3 boys are at school. My sweet friend Wendy, who is SO cute and a crafty type, created a book of "Comfort Scriptures" for me. Every page is a different scrapbook-page background and a scripture that gives God's promise to those who are sick, weak, weary, and troubled. So many verses seemed to jump out at me, but here's one that was particularly special (obvious adjustments mine):

> "Because Allyson loves me," says the Lord, "I will rescue her; I will protect her, for she acknowledges My name. She will call upon Me, and I will answer her; I will be with her in trouble, I will deliver her and honor her." (Psalm 91:14–15)

I claim this verse not just in relation to my illness, but for my day-to-day life. Here's how the week has gone, and how the Father kept His promise: Mom went home and Hubs went back to work. Still unable to do virtually anything, and still in pain, I definitely needed rescuing! So I started making phone calls. The end result? A beautiful orchestration of different people meeting very real needs. God sent Hope, Jennifer, and Bethany to cook for us. He gave us Kelly, who has provided Goliath his own personal school bus (complete with a juice box each afternoon) and a new friend in her sweet little girl. He nudged Theresa, Heather, Cassie, and John in our direction to help with endless hours of childcare so that Mommy can rest. He opened the hearts of my fellow teachers/friends, who gifted us a clean house! There are so many more who continue to call or come by just to check on us, or make grocery runs for the milk we're always out of, or show special affection to our boys, or minister to us in a million other ways. There is no way I can feel anything less than loved and honored! Now...a special shout out to our friends in the Houston area. Many of you we don't even know, but we are well-acquainted with the gifts of grace and love that you've given to us. The tangible ways you love us turn up in our mailbox almost every day—cards, small gifts, flowers, notes of encouragement. The things we don't see—when you are loving on our family there, or when you are on your knees praying for us—matter even more. Thank you. It has been 2 weeks since Surgery 2, and we are still waiting on pathology reports to confirm or refute what Dr. M did not find. I will see him for follow-up on Monday. Please pray that he has those reports in hand when we walk in. It feels like my whole life is in a holding pattern while we wait. May your weekend be blessed with beautiful weather and time well spent with loved ones. My boys are goin' fishing!

Results

Monday, September 17, 2007

> This is the confidence we have in approaching God: that if we ask anything according to His will, He hears us. And if we know that He hears us—whatever we ask—we know that we have what we asked of Him. (1 John 5:14–15)

GOD HAS HEARD US AND answered our prayer. I saw my oncologist today and was declared to be CANCER FREE!!! During Surgery 2 (2 1/2 weeks ago), the only cancer to be found was in the remaining ovary, which was removed as part of the hysterectomy. There were no cancer cells in any of my lymph nodes or on any other organs. No further treatment is necessary: no chemotherapy, no radiation. Dr. M only requires an exam in November, and scans every 6 months after that. He advised me to walk out of his office and walk back into my life, and to tell my children that their mom will live to be an old lady. There is much celebrating going on in our four walls today. Make no mistake—cancer will always be part of my life. But today I was transformed from cancer patient to cancer survivor. My mom and I were talking on the way to DSW Shoes this afternoon (doesn't every survivor need a great pair of shoes?), and here's what we agree on: Even if the results were different...if I had gone in this morning and learned my body was ravaged by deadly cancer cells and there were only months left to live on this earth...God would still be God. He would still be good, still be loving, still be merciful. He would still be in control of my life; He would still sit on His throne. I have seen the power of God today, and I will never be the same.

> Shout with joy to God, all the earth! Sing the glory of His name, make His praise glorious! Say to God, "How awesome are your deeds! So great is your power!"...Come and see what God has done!" (Psalm 66:1–5)

New Year, Fresh Start

Monday, October 15, 2007

TODAY IS MY BIRTHDAY. THIS day each year is special, but it seems that the older I get (and the more kids I have) it is less significant and not as celebrated. Not so this year. This morning dawned dark and rainy, but I feel as though the sun is shining through every window. Knowing that had things gone differently, this birthday could have very well been my last—or I might not have seen it at all—has changed me. God not only spared my life but gave me a new outlook as well. I am grateful for the time I have and I intend to spend it well. I am so thankful for my family: my 4 guys love me and gave me a reason to fight to get well. I am blessed with the greatest friends a girl could ask for. I may not understand why God allowed me to endure the trial of cancer, but I understand that the lessons to be learned from my experience are a treasure. It is my prayer that the coming year will be filled with "ah-ha!" moments, when I catch a glimpse of the Father's amazing plan for me, side-splitting laughter, and tremendous love.

P.S. Here are my 3 little cowboys, picnicking in the backyard last week:

This One's for You, Kandice...

Friday, December 07, 2007

IT HAS BEEN BROUGHT TO my attention that I am doing a poor job at keeping up with the blog. So, just in case you're one of those who is faithfully checking in, here's what we've been up to the last few weeks:

1. I gave my testimony at our church's Thanksgiving dinner. I totally get why Moses felt like he needed Aaron, as I am no public speaker myself. But my prayer has been that God would "enlarge my territory," so I had to take advantage of this opportunity. Perhaps I will post what I said on 3littlecowboys sometime soon.
2. Hubby went out of town and I came down with a delightful flu/strep throat combo Thanksgiving week. My mom and sister saved the day when they drove from Houston to Dallas and back in one day to collect my kids so I could rest. I spent 3 yucky (but quiet!) days in bed.
3. Hubby and I traveled to Houston for Thanksgiving. We ate a delicious meal, spent sweet time with our family—including my brother, who made the trip from

Nashvegas—, and made a quick departure when all 3 boys came down with pink eye. In spite of incessant handwashing and sanitizing, Nana caught it from them. Sorry, Nana.

4. The moment we returned from Houston, we began decorating our home for Christmas. I was so happy to see our pre-lit tree we bought last year!!! The boys love decorating the tree. When it was all said and done, we had very few ornaments on the upper half of the tree, and several branches were sagging because they held more than one ornament. I wanted to "fix" it after the boys went to bed, but Hubs reminded me that it will only look this way for a few short years. We left it as it was, and they are so proud.

5. I had visits with both my ob-gyn and my oncologist. Hormones (or lack thereof) are taking a toll, but I have been assured that there's nothing wrong with me that is not wrong with many other women, though they may be 20+ years my senior. Supposedly the right combination of medications can make me cheerful and whole again. We're working on that. I will be scheduled for a CAT scan in January to begin the cycle of searching for returning cancer. My oncologist kissed me on the head.

6. We had visits from two of our favorite families in Abilene. It was a fun day of eating and catching up. Happy Birthday, Jared and Tyler!!!

7. Our family was asked to light an Advent candle during the Hanging of the Green service at church. If you've ever taken a 2-year-old to "big church" you know where this is headed… I let Baby read the hymnal, sit with assorted friends, and even fed him goldfish (although I have a rule that the kids can NEVER eat in church) to keep him quiet. It was finally our turn to light the candle, and when I picked him up to walk to the stage, his shoe fell

off. I carried him down front with only one shoe on, and the whole time he was yelling, "SHOE! SHOE! SHOE, MAMA!!!!" Serene and holy we were NOT.

8. Baby moved to a big boy bed. He is SO proud, and when he woke up after the first night in it, he said to me, "I big, Mama." I cried. We loaned the crib—which has been used constantly for nearly 6 years—to some friends, and I cried. Babyhood is no more at my house!
9. We got a new oven. That's the good news. The bad news is that the new oven is bigger than the old oven. I spent 2 days this week at home listening to the sounds of new cabinetry being manufactured in my garage. Everything I own was covered in sawdust.
10. After a little holiday hiatus, the lady who cleans my house came back today. The sawdust is gone and I am happy. And there you have it. Thanks for the gentle nudge, KC!

More Medical Mishaps

Friday, January 11, 2008

POOR BABY.

Today he had his 3rd (count 'em…3!) set of tubes put in his ears and his adenoids removed. He has a long, sad history of ear infections, so we are no strangers to the world of pediatric surgery. Taking out his adenoids was a last resort, but with 2 infections in less than a month, we knew it had to be done.

I got up at 5 a.m., made myself presentable, woke Baby up and arrived at the surgery center by 6:30. Hubby stayed home to take care of Goliath and Little Middle. Baby was SO good and sweet. He never asked for anything to eat or drink (forbidden before the procedure) or complained about being out and about so early in the morning. Once we were checked in and moved to a pre-op room, the World's Friendliest Nurse came by with a godsend: a portable DVD player and a stack of movies. Wanna guess what Baby picked?

Hola! Soy Dora. I am the most cheerfully annoying, yet captivating, animated creature the 3-and-under crowd has ever known!

Seriously. It was the best thing that could have happened this morning. He sat in a little chair and never took his eyes off the screen. Nurses came in and out, took his vital signs, asked me questions, even gave him nose spray. He barely moved. When it came time for him to go to the OR, the nurse simply scooped him up in one arm, carried DVR Dora in the other, and my son didn't look back.

Surgery took only about 20 minutes. Turns out that was the easy part. The hard part came in the recovery room. Poor little guy. He was confused and I could tell he was hurting. He was kicking hard, trying to dislodge the IV from his foot. He slept for a couple of minutes, then woke up screaming. By the time it was all said and done, he was crying, I was crying, and I'm surprised the nurse (who was expecting her first child...a boy) was not crying. Baby refused to take even a sip of juice, and he had nothing but distaste for a popsicle. The rule is that the child has to be fully hydrated before they can be released to go home. After enough screaming and carrying on, the tired nurse finally just let us go. Baby stopped crying the minute we walked out into the sunshine.

He and I took a nap when we got home while Daddy ran to the pharmacy and filled the prescriptions. Baby is on strong pain meds! We will lay low for the weekend and hopefully he will be feeling much better soon.

In other medical news, I am facing another surgery of my own. If you've been reading this for any length of time, you know what I've been through, and you also know I can't make this stuff up! :) The initial pain I had that sent me to the ER back in the summer—the visit that started the whole cancer thing—turned out to be a gallbladder attack. I have had several attacks since then, so it must come out. I have been assured that even if things go awry, the surgery (and recovery time) will be nothing like what I went through a few months ago.

Allyson Hendrickson

Goliath is going to the eye doctor for the first time tomorrow. No worries, really…just given his mama's eyesight, we'd like to be cautious.

And, last but not least, Abby Dog seems to have sprained her ankle. Do dogs have ankles? Pinched a nerve. Something. She is limping and I am sad. Hubs (aka the Dog Whisperer) is positive there is nothing broken, nothing that a little rest and lots of Scooby Snacks can't fix.

I'm off to administer medication and watch Dora reruns.

Here

Tuesday, January 29, 2008

I AM HERE. I AM not living off the illusion that there are lots of folks lurking out there, waiting for me to update my blog. I do know that there are some who check in from time to time, so it is for you that I just want to say: I am here. The birthday party went great. In spite of chilly weather, the bounce house was a hit and the boys had a good time. Goliath and his buddies partied hard and went to bed early. Good times. My gallbladder came out without much to-do. We had a bit of a scare when the doctor found a suspicious spot on my stomach, which he cut out and sent off for biopsy. Turns out it was only scar tissue and we are thankful. While I'm still moving kind of slowly and sore, this surgery almost seems like no big deal. I have lots of random thoughts running through my head about friendship… old people…church life…motherhood…people with big egos… true love. I simply don't have the energy tonight to get into all that. I am just here. And now I am leaving from here to go to bed. Although I don't think that too many people read this, I am CERTAIN that a few extra *zzzzz*'s are in order tonight. Living without my gallbladder makes me tired.

Random Reflections

Thursday, April 24, 2008

You know how we all go through dry spells in our spiritual life and/or in our relationships with other people? Where you don't feel like you have the time or the energy to put into making it as great as it could be? I've had a dry spell with my blog. Hopefully it's over and I'm ready to get back to it. Here's a bit of randomness to catch you up on the last few weeks: First, a couple of major things. Right before Spring Break, the Director of Children's Ministries at our church resigned. She talked to me about taking the position, and I said, "No, thank you." The personnel committee asked me to consider it. I said, "No, thank you." I kept saying no, but I knew I couldn't wash my hands of it without talking to God about it. So I asked Him. He directed me to Luke 9:57–62. Go ahead and read it, but I'll summarize it for you. It's the story of when Jesus is walking to Jerusalem and he says to a man, "Follow Me." The man (basically) says, "Sure, I'll follow you, but first I have to go home and tend to my dying dad." Jesus comes across another man and commands, "Follow Me." And the guy says, "Sure thing. You go on ahead and I'm just going to run home to grab a few things and say goodbye…" Here's what the author or

Three Little Cowboys

my devotional book says: "Our commitment to follow Him is more than a promise to do His will when our circumstances are right, or when His plans do not interfere with our own. It must first be to the person of Jesus Christ, even before a particular task. Total commitment...does mean Christ must be in His rightful place for everything else in our lives to be in their rightful places." I shared this with my husband, and with his encouragement and blessing, I took the job. Now I am up to my ears in Vacation Bible School, but I am excited about what the future holds for our church and our children. I had a CT scan last week. It's the first time I've been back to the Dallas hospital since November. I was dreading having it done, but it was already past time. So I put on a brave face and went. Let me just say, I am envious of people who have never had to drink that pre-test stuff. No matter what "flavor" you choose, it's awful! There's no point in rehashing the details of the scan. The combination of the terrible drink, the contrast injection, and the moving table always makes me nauseous, this time to the extreme. Skip ahead a few days... my oncologist's assistant called me last night to let me know that they don't see anything on the scan and

I am ALL CLEAR!!! Those words lifted a heavy weight from my shoulders. I am so thankful for God's protection. I face a few more tests in the next few weeks—no big deal—and I see Dr. M next week. I am much more lighthearted about it now that I know all is well. Goliath is playing baseball. This is our family's first experience with organized sports, so it's kind of a big deal. He is SO CUTE in his uniform!!! Of course, we WOULD be on the team that has to wear white pants. You moms of little boys, can I get some sympathy?!? Hubby is enjoying his undershirts being truly bright and white now because whatever goes in with the baseball pants is bleached!!! Anyway, I had really tried to talk Goliath into playing soccer. He is a lot like me in that he doesn't want to attract unwanted attention, and I thought if he played soccer he would be less likely to be singled out if it didn't go well.

Allyson Hendrickson

We "discussed" it at great length, and when it came down to it, He. Wanted. To. Play. BASEBALL. Okay then. So the first few games were rough, but now the team is kind of in the groove and they are actually doing OK. When you get a bunch of six-year-olds on the ballfield, it's really to everyone's advantage that they don't keep score. Goliath "made a score" (that's kindergartenese for "scored a run") last Saturday, and he hit a double at last night's game. His coach is impressed with his power hitting. We think that Baby tried to give himself a haircut. Or else one of the brothers helped him. Our hairdresser was mortified when we took him in earlier this week. Little Middle is definitely all boy in that he loves bugs, lizards, and all other things creepy-crawly. For his birthday, my in-laws gave him one of those caterpillar-to-butterfly kits. You get a couple of jars with live caterpillars in them and you get to watch them form their chrysalis, live in their cocoons, and transform into butterflies. Perfect gift for Little Middle! Last week the butterflies finally started emerging, and now we have a total of 8. Turns out butterflies only have a life span of 2–4 weeks (who knew?) and so we have tried to explain to him that we need to let them go soon. He's in no hurry, though, to free his pets. I cringe when

I think of what it will be like if the butterflies perish at the hands of my son! My Bible Study group met at my house this week. It was the day that we had 5 hair appointments and 2 dental cleanings, so the meal I prepared for my friends was a simple taco salad. For dessert, I made a new recipe, and it turned out so fabulous, I thought I would include it here. Girls, this is for you: Sopapilla Cheesecake 2 cans crescent rolls 3 packages cream cheese, softened 2 cups sugar, divided 1 1/2 T vanilla 1 tsp cinnamon 1 stick butter Preheat oven to 350. Beat cream cheese 1 1/2 cups sugar and vanilla until creamy. Grease 9x13 pan. Cover bottom of pan with one can crescent rolls. Spread cream cheese mixture over rolls. Top with other can. Pour melted butter over top. Combine remaining sugar and cinnamon. Sprinkle over butter. Bake for 35–40 minutes. YUM! Now, a big shout out to my friend Lisa ("Horton, this is Who. I'm in Whoville. Can you hear me?" HA!). Your poor husband's crummy work hours worked out great for me! We had a blast with you guys! You are a precious lady and I am just delighted that you are in my life. Goliath rode home hunched over in the backseat because he was worried that someone might see his near-naked, mud-covered self!!! :) My boys and I are already looking forward to next time… Tomorrow morning Hubby (who by the grace of God was spared having to travel to Los Angeles today) will come to preschool to admire Little Middle's and Baby's hard work in the annual Art Show. The kids are so proud that their stuff is on display—it's a hoot! This weekend my parents and my sister are driving up for Goliath's baseball game, followed by the elementary school's carnival on Saturday afternoon. Whew! I don't know how I'll manage it when all 3 boys are playing games and doing "stuff"! This is long and I am done. Faithful readers…consider yourself caught up!

Anniversary

Saturday, August 09, 2008

TODAY I AM CELEBRATING AN anniversary. One year ago today, I was diagnosed with ovarian cancer. (You can read about the diagnosis and the cancer journey in my archives, beginning with the August 15, 2007 post.) In many ways, this year has been the longest and most difficult of my life. In a few smaller ways, it's hard to believe that 12 months have already gone by! A cancer diagnosis—a death sentence to many—may seem like an odd thing to celebrate. But I made a promise to myself that I will never again allow August 9 to pass without reflection on what happened and celebration of my miracle. As part of my personal celebration, I pulled out the "speech" (if you want to call it that) that I gave at our church Thanksgiving dinner last year, and now I want to share it here. Names have been changed—obviously—because you just can't put every detail on the internet! :) Imagine me armed with nothing but a bunch of nerves and a small sonogram photograph. I shared this with my church family on November 11, 2007—3 months after my initial diagnosis: "Then He got into the boat and his disciples followed him. Without warning, a furious storm came up on the lake, so that the waves swept over the boat. But Jesus was sleeping. The disciples went and woke him, saying, "Lord, save us! We're going to drown!" He replied, "You of little faith, why are you so afraid?" Then he got up and rebuked the wind and the waves, and it was completely calm."

If you don't know me, you may have heard about me and perhaps even prayed for me. My name is Allyson. I am a daughter, a sister, a friend, a teacher, and most importantly, I am a wife and a mommy. This account from the Bible could just as well describe the last few months of my life.

This summer I was enjoying my sons, especially savoring the last weeks before Goliath would start kindergarten. On the morning of June 30, I woke up feeling a pain in my back I had never had before. The pain intensified to the point I thought I was having a heart attack. Aimee came over and drove me to the hospital. 12 hours and 4 scans later, I was released with no definite diagnosis, but a warning that there was a mass on my left ovary and I should make an appointment with my doctor. I did so, and she determined that it was probably nothing to worry about, but it would be a good idea to remove it. Surgery was scheduled for August 7.

The operation went smoothly. I really wasn't worried about much except the time it would take me to recover. Then, on August 9, Dr. A came in for her morning rounds. My mom was with me to hear the six words that would change my life forever: "I have bad news. It's cancer." I don't remember much after that except calling Hubby. He came right away, and we all cried together.

One week later I sat in an oncologist's office. Although I'd been assured he was the best around, I was very nervous and uncomfortable. He explained the components of my cancer, admitted that it appeared to have spread some, and advised that I undergo another surgery as soon as possible to remove all cancer cells and do further exploration. I spent the next week making arrangements and having pre-op work done. During that short time, Hubby and I made the heartbreaking decision to have a full hysterectomy done. We had talked about having another baby, but the risks to my health were now too great and it was not really much of a choice.

I also asked God for wisdom and courage as I told my children that their mommy was sick. I have no doubt that the Lord sat in my living room on that hot summer afternoon. I was prepared for the worst, but they only asked one question: "Mommy, are you going to get well?" The answer had to be YES.

The time leading up to my second surgery was the most difficult for me. I repeatedly asked God, "Why me?," as if He might have forgotten how young I am, or how many children I have, or how full my life is. I was scared that the surgery would not be successful. I was scared that I would have to go through chemotherapy. Mostly, I was scared that I might not live to see my sons grow up to be men. My prayers were filled with questions and tears as I asked God for a miracle. Slowly—almost without my noticing—my fear was replaced with peace.

On August 30, 2 months after my ER visit, I was back in an OR. Dr. M removed all visible signs of cancer and performed the hysterectomy. Hours later, I began to come out of the fog of anesthesia and saw my entire family gathered around my bed. Hubby said to me, "They got it all. There is no more cancer," and we cried together again.

Recovery has been painful and very slow. Those first weeks after surgery I was fully dependent on other people to do everything for me. I couldn't take care of my home or my children. Though I desperately wanted to feel "normal" I was unable to do much more than lay in bed. Plus, I was burdened with the possibility that the biopsies and other tests might still reveal bad news. On the day of my follow-up appointment, I was a nervous wreck. The doctor came in almost immediately, seeming nearly cheerful. He said that all tests showed that the cancer was fully removed, had not spread, and that I should go home and start living my life again. My God had calmed the storm, and I had received my miracle.

If God had chosen to work in a different way—to allow the cancer to spread, or for me to go through treatments, or even to take my life—He would still be God. He had all my days laid out for me before I was even born. My mom tells of the moment it became clear for her: When I was waiting on a gurney to be wheeled to the operating room for the second surgery, she placed her hands on my stomach where the cancer hid. She thought of how Abraham was willing to sacrifice his son, Isaac, because it was what God asked of him. For the rest of my family, this journey has been that life-changing. We have come face to face with the power and the true character of God, knowing that my purpose is only to glorify my Father. He is unchanging, He is faithful, He is sovereign. I may never understand why He allowed this storm of cancer to surround me, but I praise Him because He would not let me drown. In my time of need, God never left his throne—He only drew me closer to it.

There is one more part of my story that not many people know. You can't see this very well from where you sit, but if you were to look closely you would see a perfectly formed, wonderfully made baby waiting to make his grand entrance into the world. He was a total surprise to his mom and dad, but not a surprise to God. This picture was taken 2 ½ years ago, and that baby is my youngest son. While I never questioned the existence of my baby, I sure did wonder about God's timing. I already had a baby at home—and a toddler—and a new baby was NOT in my plan until much later. My plan was flawed, though, and God's plan was perfect. He knew what lay ahead for me. He knew that if we didn't have Baby in the fall of 2005, we would never have had Baby at all. Today is Baby's 2nd birthday. Every morning when he calls my name as he wakes up, or when he runs into my arms, or when he climbs up on my lap to read a book, I am reminded that my God is indeed an awesome God. His ways are not our ways, nor His thoughts our thoughts…and I am thankful.

All I Need

Friday, November 21, 2008

I will lift my eyes to the hills—from whence comes my help? My help comes from the Lord, who made heaven and earth. He will not allow your foot to be moved; He who keeps you will not slumber. (Psalms 121:1–3)

For I am the Lord your God, who takes hold of your right hand and says to you, "Do not fear, I will help you." (Isaiah 41:13)

Cancer Scare Timeline

Tuesday, November 25, 2008

THURSDAY MORNING: Went for a regular check-up with my oncologist. He determined that a combination of factors warranted testing to check for returning cancer. Did a blood test in the office and gave them the "best number to reach me at." Put on a brave face and tried to ignore the panic welling up inside.

THURSDAY AFTERNOON: Played with my kids. Wondered how I would tell them their mommy has cancer—again. Remembered the power of my miracle and realized that nothing is impossible with God.

FRIDAY MORNING: Stood in a circle of my friends and co-workers as they approached the throne boldly on my behalf. Cried. Looked around and was amazed to see so many of them in tears as well.

FRIDAY AFTERNOON: Received a call that the CA-125 was normal. Didn't really believe it because I had the same results in July '07, and they were wrong. Returned a call from the hospital and was surprised to be able to schedule the CT scan for the next morning.

Allyson Hendrickson

SATURDAY MORNING: Dropped off a dozen donuts, a quart of chocolate milk, and my 3 boys at Shannon's house. Said a prayer thanking God for such a great friend and asking him to preserve her sanity while I was gone. Drove to the hospital. Spent 3 hours drinking barium, praying I wouldn't get sick, and doing the scan and x-rays. Left there relieved it was over and asking God for clear scans. Picked up my kids.

SATURDAY AFTERNOON: Went to see Madagascar 2. Fell asleep in Madagascar 2. Promised myself I'd go to bed early.

SUNDAY: Went to church. Hosted a playdate for Goliath. Tried hard to conquer Mount Laundry. Took a gift to a friend who just lost her mom. Got perspective. Took the boys to Awana.

MONDAY: Got a phone call: ALL CLEAR. Wept with relief and gratitude. Called my Hubby. Rejoiced together. Called everyone else. Got busy preparing to really celebrate Thanksgiving.

> When I said, "My foot is slipping," your love, O Lord, supported me. When anxiety was great within me, your consolation brought joy to my soul. (Psalm 94:18–19)

Out with the Old, In with the New

Thursday, January 01, 2009

IN 2008, I...

- had gallbladder surgery.
- witnessed a baby cow being born, WAY up close.
- forgave—but will never forget—Hubby setting the kitchen on fire, and the subsequent long-term flooring project.
- became a baseball mom.
- lost my Grandad to cancer.
- celebrated 10 years of marriage with my one-and-only. Babe, I love you!
- beamed with pride as my first-born graduated from kindergarten.
- made fantastic memories with my family on our vacation to Disneyland.
- survived my first earthquake, and hung Hubby's Associated Press article on the fridge.
- spent a fabulous summer in the sun, having fun with my boys.

- celebrated 1 year of being cancer-free!
- shared deep sorrow, great joy, and one really fun weekend with my Tuesday night sisters.
- experienced God's hand of protection during another cancer scare.
- thoroughly enjoyed a sweet time in Houston with my dad who played board games (?!?!?), my sister who is a new graduate with a bright future, my brother who has found tremendous healing and restoration, and my mom who has her Christmas groove back.
- spent my first Christmas at home and cooked my first-ever Christmas dinner.

I opened my eyes this morning to the first day of 2009. Happy New Year! I try not to make New Year's resolutions…I tend to set goals that are beyond the boundaries of the time, willpower, or ambition I have. It's a sure bet for failure—no thank you. Instead, I like to think about the new year in a general terms. 2008 was overall a good year (anything beats '07!). There's always room for improvement, though, so here are a few things I will be working toward:

1. Simplifying
2. Quality, not quantity
3. Richness and depth in my relationships
4. True gratitude for life's blessings
5. Knowing God in a fresh, new way Happy New Year!

Wow.

Friday, April 03, 2009

God's love is meteoric, His loyalty astronomic, His purpose titanic, His verdicts oceanic. Yet in His largeness nothing gets lost; Not a man, not a mouse, slips through the cracks. How exquisite Your love, O God! Psalm 36:5–7a, The Message

Today in Bible Study...

Sunday, April 05, 2009

I ASKED FOR HEALTH THAT I might do great things, I was given infirmity that I might do better things. I asked for riches that I might be happy, I was given poverty that I might be wise. I asked for power, that I might have the praise of men, I was given weakness, that I might feel the need for God. I asked for all things, that I might enjoy life; I was given life, that I might enjoy all things. I got nothing I asked for, but everything I hoped for. Almost despite myself, my unspoken prayers were answered. I am, among all men, most richly blessed. Unknown Confederate Soldier

He Lives!

Sunday, April 12, 2009

On the first day of the week, very early in the morning, the women took the spices they had prepared and went to the tomb. They found the stone rolled away from the tomb, but when they entered, they did not find the body of the Lord Jesus. While they were wondering about this, suddenly two men in clothes that gleamed like lightning stood beside them. In their fright the women bowed down with their faces to the ground, but the men said to them, "Why do you look for the living among the dead? He is not here; he has risen!" (Luke 24:1–6)

My Heart Cries

Thursday, June 11, 2009

I've been in a funk lately. I could attribute it to a few things: the endless deluge of laundry and other household drudgery, the start of summer (my least favorite of the seasons), the plywood covering the hole in our living room ceiling where part of the air conditioner leaked, the heat. But the funk came to a head a few days ago and it was time to get honest. I recently made my bi-annual visit to my oncologist (it's amazing how quickly those six months go by!). The appointment was routine—nothing out of the ordinary, nothing that raised any extra concerns. He applauded my efforts at fitness and weight loss, said they would call me to schedule CT scans, and sent me on my way. Don't get me wrong—Dr. M is a nice guy. He saved my life. But even that does not endear me to him or get me excited about seeing him in that awful, pastel office where sickness sits on every surface and desperation lingers in the air. That office visit was followed a few days later by a party! One of my Bible Study besties is having a baby, and we gathered to celebrate. We had so much fun ooohing and aaahing over the gifts, eating cake, and laughing at Amilee's pregnancy craving—french toast. She will be a great mom. But when I got home that afternoon, I felt dejected and sadder than I've felt in a long time. Hubby called me out on it, asking for—and deserving—an explanation. What's wrong with me is that I miss what I can't have. Two years ago, six words turned our world upside down: "I have bad news. It's cancer." That moment is etched in my memory forever. The months that followed were difficult as I underwent treatment, but I was eventually deemed to be cancer-free and encouraged to resume life as normal. And for the most part, I have learned to live with my new "normal." Normal now includes those doctor visits and trips to a hospital for scans on a regular basis. Normal means that I pay close attention to my body, fighting the urge to worry that a headache could be a brain tumor or abdominal pain is more than cramps. Normal for me is battling fear and having an oncologist's number programmed into my phone. And normal means letting go. In order to eliminate existing cancer and as a preventative measure for future reoccurrences, we were given the "option" to have a full hysterectomy performed. It wasn't really much of a choice! Kids or cancer. Wow. It was a no-brainer to know that I wanted to be around for a long, long time to raise my boys up to be men. But before cancer tore its way into our lives, I had other plans in mind for raising my children. I wanted more of them! Standing in my kitchen, sobbing in my husband's arms, I confessed how angry I am that the chance for more children was ripped away from me. I told him that I mourn the baby that will never be. I affirmed my complete love and total devotion to him and our three boys. I asked him why I can't have peace about this. I admitted that I recognize the sin of discontent and ungratefulness and I feel guilty for it. I dismissed his comfort and his invitation to hang out in his man-cave! I swam in self-pity, right there in my own kitchen. Many people I know—close friends, not-so-close friends, co-workers, moms of the boys' friends—are expecting or have recently welcomed new babies. Again, don't misunderstand me. I am happy for those families and want to celebrate each little baby! How blessed am I that I got to bring three new lives into this world?!? Those three tiny blue bundles have brought tremendous love and joy into our home, only to expand as they grow. My heart longs to add on, and I just can't. My life was threatened by a disease that grabbed hold of my body and my family without me even knowing it! The events that led to the discovery of the sickness came straight from God's hand, no doubt about it. The treatment and medical care I received were quality, and much less invasive than what so many other cancer patients endure. I know I should feel gratitude. Believe me…I KNOW. And I DO. But my life changed with six words. That change didn't end when the surgery was over. I will always have cancer in my life. And what I had to give up for cancer still hurts.

Two Years

Sunday, August 30, 2009

You are the God who performs miracles; You display your power among the peoples. (Psalm 77:11–14)

Praise the Lord, O my soul; all my inmost being, praise His holy name. Praise the Lord, O my soul, and forget not all His benefits—who forgives all your sins and heals all your diseases, who redeems your life from the pit and crowns you with love and compassion, who satisfies your desires with good things so that your youth is renewed like the eagle's. (Psalm 103:1–5)

Two years ago today, my oncologist told me that there was no more cancer in my body, and that I should go home and tell my boys that their mama would live to be an old lady. On that day I made a promise to God: I promised that I would never let August 30th go by without remembering and celebrating the gift of His miracle. "I will remember the deeds of the Lord; yes, I will remember your miracles. I will meditate on all your works and consider all your mighty deeds. Your ways, O God, are holy. What God is so great as our God?

Allyson Hendrickson

I have this amazing circle of friends, and today they helped me celebrate! Kelly threw a "No Cancer Party" at her house. In case you're wondering what one does at a No Cancer Party…it involves dessert, heartfelt sharing, and tears. The party accomplished two things: 1) I left feeling incredibly loved, and 2) our God was given the glory and the credit He is due for what He has done!

These friends of mine…they shared their hearts, and I love them for that. I love the challenge to pray big and expect miracles. I love that my experience is theirs, too, and that we are all better Christ-followers because of my cancer.

We only get one go-round, and we're not promised anything except that we have a Savior who walks every step with us. I want this miracle-life of mine to matter, and when it's over—five years from now or fifty—I want to hear, "Well done, good and faithful servant." I choose to remember, to celebrate, and to get on with living.

"How can I repay the Lord for all His goodness to me? I will lift up the cup of salvation and call on the name of the Lord. I will fulfill my vows to the Lord in the presence of all His people." Psalm 116:12–14

P.S. After the No Cancer Party, I came home to this: Blessed, and so very, very thankful.

Safe

Sunday, February 07, 2010

ALMOST TWO WEEKS AGO, I spent a long morning in a Dallas hospital doing my bi-annual CT scan. I dread going; I am relieved to the point of tears when it's done. Five days after the test, I couldn't take the waiting anymore, so I called my oncologist's nurse. She returned my call later that day and said these words: "There are no abnormal masses, but…"

It appears that there is pelvic fluid accumulating due to an increased thickening in the mesenteric region in my upper abdomen. She was quick to point out that it could be caused by any number of things. The "C" word hung between us on the phone line like a dark cloud. She didn't say it, but I sure was thinking it.

The next day, the nurse called me again. She said that Dr. M had reviewed the images from the scan, and wanted to schedule me for a PET scan. The PET scan is a more sophisticated test, and will produce more exact images of my insides. Any "questionable" cells will "light up like a Christmas tree!" after I am injected with radioactive material.

I am waiting to find out exactly when the scan will be. Turns out my little test comes with a hefty price tag, and the guy who writes the checks at the insurance company may need to be persuaded.

I've had all sorts of thoughts and emotions, not the least of which is fear. Fear of the unknown. Fear of the next phone call. Fear of what could happen. Fear of the test. I love this quote from Beth Moore: "Christ is never intimidated by the depth of our need and the demonstration of our weakness. I'm so glad I don't have to keep a stiff upper lip and set a good example for others to follow when I am all alone with God and hurting!" I'm so glad, too.

It was during some alone time with God this weekend that an answer "accidentally" came to me through music. I wrote the lyrics of this song down in my journal this morning. That way, regardless of how this thing turns out, I can go back and remember that I learned (again) that I don't have to be afraid.

Because I am safe.

"So do not fear, for I am with you; do not be dismayed, for I am your God. I will strengthen you and help you; I will uphold you with my righteous right hand." Isaiah 41:10

Chapter 2

Wednesday, February 24, 2010

I HAVE HAD THOUSANDS OF really great days in my life. Joyous events stand out in my mind…holidays with my grandparents, graduations, the night a scavenger hunt led me to a diamond ring and a marriage proposal, my wedding day, the day I got to tell Hubby that he was going to be a daddy, the births of each of our sons. For the most part, each day is a happy one and I go to bed at night satisfied that I am very, very blessed. Yesterday, however, was not one of those days. Yesterday was the day that we had to tell our children that their mommy has cancer. Again. I would give up every single one of my good-day memories if it meant that I could have kept yesterday from happening. Forever etched in my mind will be the swollen-from-crying-green eyes of my oldest son as he looked at me and said, "Mommy, please don't die." Tomorrow I will go back to the operating room. The plan is for my oncologist to remove the 2 tumors that are growing in my abdominal cavity and on my colon, to apply intraoperative chemotherapy, and then to insert a port for post-surgery chemo access. My heart is torn, and my emotions are raw. I am scared. I am angry. I am thankful. I am still blessed. A lot of things will change for me in the coming days. I will be sick, I will be weak. I will not be able to attend Goliath's scout meetings or to cheer for my 5-year-old karate kid from the sidelines. I won't teach preschool, I won't do much cooking, and I will not take Baby to the library. But in the midst of my heartache, my God remains the same. He was faithful before, and I believe He will be faithful again. I wish so much that I could understand why I must endure this. Little Middle asked me yesterday, "Mommy, why do you have to have cancer?" The answer could only be, "I don't know why God lets bad things happen to good people." But I do know that the God who gave me those three precious boys holds me and my cancer in the palm of His hand. And knowing that I am safe there is enough to make today a better day.

> Because of the Lord's great love we are not consumed, for his compassions never fail. They are new every morning; GREAT IS YOUR FAITHFULNESS. (Lamentations 3:22–23)

3 Days and Counting

Sunday, February 28, 2010

After a restless night, I woke up to the cheerfulness of my daytime nurse proclaiming, "It's Sunday!"

Sunday means that I have been in the hospital for three days. I expect to be here for at least two more.

Sunday means that I get to try a clear liquid diet. I haven't had anything to eat or drink since Thursday.

Sunday means that I get to take a shower! I am looking pretty rough.

Sunday means that God's people are gathering together in God's house. I am missing it.

The cancer is back, more abundant and aggressive than we first thought. I wish I were at church meeting with God this morning instead of in this hospital room trying to make sense of Him.

Day 4

Monday, March 01, 2010

I AM WAKING UP THIS morning to a cold rain falling outside my window. Today is the 4th day after my surgery to remove cancer from my body and prepare for chemo. In spite of where I am and what I'm facing, a few good things happened over the weekend:

- My 3 little cowboys came to see me! Hospital policy prohibits children under the age of 12 from visiting (due to the flu threat, we're told). However, my daytime nurse was kind and very compassionate, and helped Hubby smuggle the little guys in. It was a sweet visit—good for them, and good for me. Goliath brought his Nintendo DS to me so I would have something to play with while I'm here.
- My room was a revolving door for my family, who took turns coming to sit (and sleep!) with me. My Hubs, my parents, Sister and her Mister, and Brother and his Other all came to visit/fetch ice chips/watch movies/watch me sleep.
- My soon-to-be-brother-in-law had "Team Allyson" bracelets made for all of us to wear. They are Lance Armstrong-style, imprinted with the words "courage,

- strength, hope, faith" and teal in color to represent ovarian cancer. I wear mine with pride.
- My dad left late last night to return to Houston, but not before we had a great talk about what's to come. In his own special way, he challenged me to pursue God through the dark and scary days. We're all frightened, we're all bewildered…but without our God, we are nothing at all.

Even as I type this, the doctor has just come in for his morning rounds. Not much change to report—everyone is holding their breath for when my body might seem ready to try real food again. I had apple juice for breakfast yesterday, and a purple popsicle for dinner. Going home seems to hinge on that.

Thank you for your continued prayers and support. We are overwhelmed by the outpouring of love that is coming from God's people. Please specifically pray that I will be able to eat soon. I haven't had "real" food since last Wednesday. Please also pray for healing of the incisions, and for my spirit as I begin to look ahead to chemotherapy. And…pray for my family. My sons seem to be handling my absence well, and I know that is only because they are so loved and prayed for. I am asking God to continue to protect them in the coming days, and to put in their path people who will be especially kind and tender with them. For my husband, as he carries the weight of the world on his shoulders. And for my mom, who is moving in to my house today to run my household and take care of my kids. There is no greater love than those two people have for me.

This is the verse my mom posted on Facebook this morning. I will borrow it because it is my truth:

> But as for me, the nearness of God is my good. (Psalm 73:28)

Day 5

Tuesday, March 02, 2010

It's been a tough day today. Yesterday, when we all prayed that my stomach and all related systems would "wake up," maybe we should have prayed for a slower awakening. A delicious dinner of Jell-O and a popsicle did the trick, but I was sick much of the night. Dr. M came in this morning and was delighted with my misery! I graduated from a clear liquid diet to an all-liquid diet…the main difference is that I can have milk-based products. Brother brought me a vanilla milkshake when he came by this morning, but I just couldn't drink much. Hubby is promising some applesauce later this afternoon. I know that eating is the ticket out of here, but today it just seems to be more than I can bear.

If I'd known I would go through all of this, I might not have been working so hard at the gym over the last few months. This is a much more time-effective weight-loss plan…

Hubby has pointed out—and he is right—that I am out of place on the 9th floor of Medical City. All of the other patients are older women whose visitors are their elderly husbands or grown children. My babies being here the other day was probably a breath of fresh air to the staff!

There is a patient down the hall who apparently does not understand how the nurse call button works. Every time she needs a nurse, she just starts hollering, "HELP! HELP! HELP!" until someone comes. People in my room think that is pretty funny.

The central line came out today. Good news: No more wires and tubes sticking out, giving me that Bride of Frankenstein look. Bad news: No more Demerol on demand.

I am weary, and my spirits are low. Please pray that I will be faithful in looking for Jesus today. And please continue to pray for the ultimate—complete healing and deliverance from this disease.

> "You pay God a compliment by asking great things of Him."
> —St. Teresa of Avila

Day 6

Wednesday, March 03, 2010

In a disappointing turn of events, we just found out that today will not be the day I get to go home. My new-found freedom to consume all liquids has gone just as quickly as it came yesterday. During the course of the day yesterday, I drank a little bit of a vanilla milkshake, ate a few spoonfuls of strawberry ice cream, took a few sips of a fruit smoothie, and had some ice chips. I felt weak and shaky for much of the day, just like you do when your blood sugar has dropped too low and you need food. I just couldn't handle more than what I had! Hubby spent the night with me last night, and I woke up early this morning with that same weak and shaky feeling. I drank a little bit of apple juice, hoping that the sugar would help with the icky feeling. No sooner had the juice gone down than it came right back up. And with that juice went my ticket home today.

The good doctor has ordered an x-ray of my belly today so they can get a clear picture of what is (or is not) happening in there. I am also set to be re-hooked to an IV line so I can be re-hydrated and will receive pain meds through that line. It is not a good feeling to take oral pain meds on an empty stomach!

In other news, my left leg is numb. The numbness started on Day 2, and has gone from total loss of feeling to tingling and back again. The doctor tells me it is most likely due to the use of a retractor during surgery, which might have pressed on a nerve. Numbness is not uncommon, and should go away on its own. Still—how annoying! It reminds me of when Baby was born and one of my legs was numb from anesthesia. When the nurses tried to help me move from one bed to another, I literally collapsed under my own weight and the nurse had to dive to catch me. Good memories.

I miss my babies. I talk to them every afternoon, and every night before bedtime. My mom and my husband tell me how good they are being…how helpful…how kind to each other…how hard they are trying. My heart breaks every time I think of them there, and me here, and how much I want to be with them.

Please pray today that the IV will do its trick. Pray that the fluids will fill my body and that I will lose that sickly feeling so that I can work on eating. I WANT TO GO HOME. Everything I do is working toward that.

Day 7

Thursday, March 04, 2010

IT HAS BEEN ONE WEEK since I entered the hospital. I never imagined I would be here this long! God has been so gracious in placing kind and caring people in my path. Every physician, nurse, orderly, and even the little lady who cleans my room each day has gone out of their way to take excellent care of me. In spite of where I am and what I'm up against, those little glimpses of God's grace are not lost on me.

So, first things first. Today will not be the day I go home. I'm starting to sound like a broken record! Yesterday's abdominal x-ray was clear and normal. It's just a matter of time for everything to come together and work like it should, or so they tell me. I enjoyed 2 more popsicles yesterday, and tried some Jell-o… have I mentioned that I don't really care for Jell-o? The clear liquid diet has been tough for me because 1) it tastes yucky, and 2) I'm not a fan of many clear-liquid items.

This morning the doctor is encouraged at my popsicle progress and I will again be graduated to an all-liquid diet. Right now, not much sounds good, but I think a vanilla milkshake will be part of the plan later today. IF today is a good day, I might be able to try solid food for breakfast/lunch tomorrow, and IF that goes well, I can possibly go home tomorrow afternoon. Those are pretty big IFs!

The second part of this post is actually a continuation of Day 6. After I posted yesterday morning, Dr. M (my oncologist) came by to tell us that the pathology reports had come back from the surgery. The news was not unexpected, but still very hard to hear. The cancer that he removed last week is actually the same ovarian cancer that we dealt with two years ago, but it had re-differentiated itself into a bigger, badder, meaner kind of a cancer. "High-level cancer" were his actual words. Dr. M was encouraged because we caught it early and he got all of the visible cancer out during surgery. He also said, however, that it is unusual for this cancer to change and come back in this way, and of course, that only adds to the frustration to the never-ending "Why Me?" question.

Then again, my sweet husband has gently pointed out...why not me? I was not promised that I will get to walk where I want—only that where I must go, He will walk with me.

"We are hard pressed on every side, but not crushed; perplexed, but not in despair; persecuted, but not abandoned; struck down, but not destroyed." 2 Corinthians 4:8

Day 8

Friday, March 05, 2010

Yesterday...

- I drank 1/2 of a vanilla milkshake, a small apple juice, and ate 1 scrambled egg, 2 saltine crackers, and 4 bites of a baked potato.
- I had my IV removed and switched back to oral pain meds.
- I walked 3.5 laps around the 9th floor.
- I started the day with stomach issues, but they tapered off and I felt pretty good by late afternoon.
- I watched Jim and Pam's baby story on The Office. Today...
- I am staying at the hospital.
- Labs were drawn to check for bacterial infection in the intestines.
- I am supposed to eat 50% more food than what I ate yesterday.
- The drain was removed from my abdomen.
- One of the daily goals that my nurse wrote on my white board is to "ambulate."
- I went downstairs to the lobby just because I finally could.

Day 9

Saturday, March 06, 2010

IT IS 4:36 P.M. GUESS what? I am posting this from my laptop while I'm sitting in MY OWN BED. Snoozing next to me is my beloved Abby dog. The sounds I'm listening to are my four guys playing Super Mario together in the next room. HOME SwEET HOME!!!

Really, not that much has changed since yesterday. I ate as much as I possibly could yesterday, but only made small dents in anything that was put in front of me. I think that having 12 inches of my colon cut out and my digestive system reconstructed is a pretty big deal—it's no wonder that nothing sounds too delicious. Lab work diffused concerns about an infection, so this morning when the doctor came in, my pleas did not fall on deaf ears. She gave me some stern warnings about what to look out for, what activities I can and can not do, who to call in case of emergency, and finally sent the nurse scurrying for discharge papers.

The greatest sight I ever saw was when Mom turned onto my street and I spotted Goliath and Little Middle riding their bikes up and down the sidewalk in front of our house. They ran to get their little brother, and the four of us shared a wonderful group hug. I didn't even care that I was wearing my pajamas for all the neighbors to see! I missed them SO MUCH…and apparently the feeling was mutual:

> Praise be to the Lord, for He has heard my cry for mercy. The Lord is my strength and my shield; my heart trusts in Him, and I am helped. My heart leaps for joy and I will give thanks to Him in song. (Psalm 28:6–7)

Laughter Is the Best Medicine

Monday, March 08, 2010

IT IS FAIR TO SAY that I have done plenty of crying over the last few weeks. My strong support system and my strong faith do not mean that I don't feel great sorrow over the disease, the treatment, or what may come in the future. I am grieving.

So it was a delightful treat last night to discover a gift that my friend Karen had left on my front porch! Karen and I met in 2006, the first year I taught at my current preschool. She was teaching 3-year-olds at the time, and her twin sons were in Goliath's class. Now, four years later, Karen and I AND our boys are still good pals. She has moved on to get a full-time teaching job—but we make up for lost time during Girls' Night Out with Mexican food and margaritas!

I enjoyed Karen's gift, and I thought you might like to enjoy it with me. The card attached to the bag said, "The Official I Love Allyson So Much That I Bought Her a Bunch Of Stuff From the Dollar Store Bag."

Here's the loot:

Want to get a closer look? OK. Each item has written below it the note that Karen attached to it:

"Made in China." Hmmmm...probably contains high levels of lead and cadmium. Enjoy!

This is a Coach knock-off. Can you believe how realistic it is?!?!?

Happy St. Patrick's Day!

Celebrity Good Life, eh? You can now hit the red carpet like a superstar! WOW! Well, at least you now have some oversized sunglasses to wear.

I got this for the message. Who knew that was all that love was? I have been doing it wrong all these years! (And don't look too close at the picture. I think more than surfing is going on.)

This says "collector's series." I sure hope this completes your "Ye Old Crappy Painted Churches of England" collection.

What every cool beverage will be wearing this spring!

Trouble eating? You just needed some "Eazee Squeeze!"

The only useful item in this bag.

You too can smell like Britney Spears! Then you can go catch butterflies.

Wow! Contains 2 packs of trading cards! You can now trade with yourself, and yourself! Nothing says "class" and "style" like nail art!

Oh...this is for you, not the boys—just to make that clear.

You will need these for the "Celebrity Good Life"... So many jokes...so little time.

One word: purple!!

In the middle of my sadness, I am SO thankful for friends who "get" me. Sick or not, I am still me. The same things still make me sad, the same things still make me laugh. This care package—and many other gifts, cards, and letters I have received this past week—have put a smile on my face. Cancer can't take that from me!

Looking for Answers

Friday, March 12, 2010

I SPENT SOME SWEET TIME yesterday with my friend Lisa. We laughed a lot—we always do—and cried a little while we discussed all things cancer. She pierced my heart when she confessed that she doesn't even know how to wrap her mind around what is happening to me, or what exactly to pray for when it comes to my sickness. I totally understand what she meant: It comes back to the crazy question that doesn't seem to have an answer: WHY? I would be dishonest if I said that I haven't had moments of anger and great sadness. I have shaken my proverbial fist at God and wondered aloud if He made a big mistake. I have read and re-read Job's story of suffering, and tried to connect the parallel dots of our lives. I have asked my husband over and over again if he can maybe see a bigger picture that I can't (he doesn't) and asked my friends and family to plead with God for healing (they are). I don't get it. I can't explain to my children, to my friends, or to anyone else why this terrible disease is invading my life because I don't know. I, too, am unable to wrap my mind around it or look far enough ahead to see what God might have in store. But I told Lisa through my tears yesterday that I don't think that

Allyson Hendrickson

God is waiting on me to be able to explain Him. I think He only wants me to trust Him. Do I honestly think that my body was stricken with cancer when God was not looking? Of course not. Do I think He was surprised on February 17th when the doctor said to us, "There is a new tumor growing?" Nope. Do I feel forgotten and unloved? No way. My Lord's love letter to me says: "All the days ordained for me were written in your book before one of them came to be." (Psalm 139:16) He knew long, long ago that cancer would be part of my life. He knew that there would be a Chapter 2. He does not need my input, my advice, or my approval. He only wants my obedience. In John chapter 9 we are told the story of the blind man. v.2: "The disciples asked him, 'Rabbi, who sinned, this man or his parents, that he was born blind?'" That's the same question so many people are asking about me and my cancer: Why did this happen? And right there, in verse 3, is the answer we are all searching for. If you don't look carefully at Jesus' red words, you might miss it: "Neither this man nor his parents sinned, but this happened so that the work of God might be displayed in his life." I am not under the illusion that my life is of any more value than any one else's. I don't think that I stand to lose more or that people would be any more affected by my sickness or even my death than any other cancer patient. Lots of women have ovarian cancer—statistically, my story is just another sad tale. But I do think that God is continually at work all around us. As Christians, we easily grow complacent and are content to look for Him when the flowers bloom in the spring, when our bank accounts swell, or when we experience success. But we are truly thankful for food when we feel hungry. We don't give much thought to wellness until we are sick. We take for granted the roofs over our heads and the clothes on our back until we are poverty-stricken. We don't give much thought to the hope and the life we've been given until we are hopeless. Maybe, just maybe, while God works, His power will be much more evident against the backdrop that none of us expected—a healthy, happy, young woman with a family to raise. I could (and probably will, at some point on this silly little blog) tell hundreds of stories of ways I have seen God work in the last three weeks. Some of them are specific answers to prayer, some of them are ways He has shown up where I didn't even know I needed Him. He has used people very close to me, and He has used absolute strangers to remind me of the very essence of the faith I stand on: He is good, and He does good. Take my life and let it be consecrated, Lord, to Thee. Take my moments and my days, let them flow in ceaseless praise, let them flow in ceaseless praise.

Today's Blog Post Is Brought to You by the Letter C

Thursday, March 18, 2010

Cowboys
Creation
Crazy
Canine Companion
Caroline
Cute
Cookies and Caring
Crying, Cancer, Chemotherapy

Wanting to Worship

Sunday, March 21, 2010

I AM SPENDING A LAZY Sunday afternoon in my polka-dot pajamas, curled up in my bed. Outside the window, I am watching the last of a Texas spring snow melt away and trying not to think about how much I enjoyed the 70 degree temperatures less than 48 hours ago. In the other room, I can hear the little cowboys cheering and jeering their way through a new Wii game. Hubby is passing back and forth, cleaning out cabinets—due in part to boredom, and in part to a need for some spring cleaning around here. He's a good, good man. This morning I got up early, got all fancied up in my best jeans, and headed to the church house. I haven't been to church in a month, and I HAVE MISSED IT. I am of the opinion that the command God gives us to "not give up meeting together" (Hebrews 10:25) is a lovely one indeed. We love our church. I was glad to be there when my boys practically skipped into their classrooms. I was glad to be there when I got hugs from friends, big and small, who I haven't seen in a while. I was glad to be there when "my" usher, Mr. Bill (who keeps mini chocolate bars in his coat pocket to give to the kids each week), opened the door for me and when I made eye contact with precious Ms. Dessie over the balcony railing and blew her a kiss. I was glad to be there to sing the words of the great hymn "Come, Thou Fount of Every Blessing." I was glad to be there to hear a sermon on what authentic worship is and what it is not. I jotted this tidbit down in my notes: "Worship is done everywhere—even in the middle of crisis and disaster." What a timely reminder! I will be mindful of that when I go back to the oncology office on Wednesday for a chemotherapy teaching session. This session, slated to last 1 1/2 hours, will be Hubby and me and my parents, learning everything we ever wanted (or did not want) to know about chemo. She will tell us when my chemo sessions will be, what to expect, and what they think the drugs will or will not do to my body. They say that information is power, but I am scared of what I will learn at that appointment. I don't want to find out about a chemotherapy protocol that has been specially designed for me. I don't even want it to exist! Even more than that, I dread what must happen after the appointment on Wednesday. Hubby and I must sit down with our sons and try to explain chemotherapy to them. I have the same knot in my stomach that I had four weeks ago when we told them that the cancer had returned. How can I explain to my children that the only way to fight is with more sickness? This seems even more complicated after a conversation I had with Goliath yesterday. He and I went out in the snow yesterday afternoon to run a few errands, and on our way back I stopped at the dry cleaners to pick up some clothes we had waiting there. It went something like this: Goliath: Mom, what are we doing here? Me: I need to pick up these sweaters so Dad has them for church tomorrow. Goliath: Why are we going to church tomorrow? Me: Ummm…because we always go to church. We haven't been able to go for a few weeks, but it's important that we are there to learn and worship. Goliath: We just didn't go because of your surgery. Me: That's right, buddy. Goliath, do you think that God stopped loving me because I got sick? Goliath: Noooooo… Me: And do you think that God stopped loving you and your brothers and your dad because you feel sad about me? Goliath: Nooooo…that's not how it works. But Mom, I don't know why we have to talk about this, because you're not sick anymore. My sons believe that I am well. They understand that I am not 100%—they see me resting and taking medicine—but as far as we can tell, they think that my release from the hospital meant that the cancer is over. This week will be a bad surprise for them. This disease is my crisis, my own personal disaster. I am sad and scared. But in spite of that, I want to worship. I want to show my sons what real worship looks like, so they can draw from that when they are ready. God is not contained by my cancer or boxed in by my sorrow. His goodness and loving kindness reach far beyond my weakness. Even when I am hurting, I will choose to worship. Streams of mercy, never ceasing, call for songs of loudest praise. He is so worthy!

> I will praise you, O Lord, with all my heart; I will tell of all your wonders. I will be glad and rejoice in you; I will sing praise to your name, O Most High. (Psalm 9:1–2)

The Thing which I Thought I Could Not Do

Tuesday, March 23, 2010

> "You gain strength, courage, and confidence by every experience in which you look fear in the face. You must do the thing which you think you cannot do."
>
> —Eleanor Roosevelt

I HAD AN EXPERIENCE LAST Thursday which I wish I could have written about last Thursday. Instead, it took me a few days to process (and cry). But I'm ready to share now…

I've mentioned here that I am pretty emotional about the possibility of losing my hair during my chemotherapy treatment. We have been told repeatedly that every patient responds differently to chemo and that every drug has different side effects. I KNOW it is possible that not a hair on my head will be lost. But a difficult situation is made a little more challenging—and beautiful—by the impending marriage of my best friend and her beloved. That wedding is close! April 17th, to be exact. I do not have the luxury of time to sit around and see if I will be one of the lucky ones. Plus, I'm not feeling exactly what you could call "lucky" these days! I keep telling Hubby that I just will prepare for the absolute worst to happen, and if we get anything besides that, it will be a pleasant surprise!

Back to the hair issue. Not only am I very, very sad about losing it; I am very, very sad that my boys will have a bald mama. My head is astronomically large—I don't think I will be a very attractive bald person. There is NO WAY that I can walk around hairless. Not for me, not for them. appointment.

So, last Thursday, my mom and my sister (who has a wedding of her own just around the corner) went with me to find a hair solution. We had contacted a shop here in the Metroplex that is run by a group of women who are all cancer survivors. In spite of my dread, we made an

Well. I thought it would be all about hair. Was I wrong! This cute little girly shop had anything and everything you could ever imagine a lady suffering through cancer might need or want. I thought nothing could make me feel happy as long as I was there, but then I saw this T-shirt:

And I laughed out loud. I might go back and buy it in a few months.

Kathy is the name of the lady who helped us. I was a mess—I cried off and on, along with Mom and Sister—almost the whole time. Kathy just talked right over the blubbering, as if my behavior was perfectly normal. She showed me what seemed like a thousand different hairstyles, colors, wigs, scarves, and hats. She spent close to two hours with me and never once strayed from kindness, compassion, and patience. She told me some of her personal story of breast cancer, but not too much. She understood when I said I'd had enough, and then she hugged me like we were old friends. Kathy promised that everything will be OK. I want so much to believe her.

As I sat there in that chair, looking at the reflection of myself wearing pretend hair, my feelings were mixed. Of course, I was sad. So very, VERY sad. But I felt just the tiniest touch of strength and pride, too. My original game plan went a little something like this: Lose hair…stay locked up in bedroom until it grows back. I was serious about it, too. BUT, I have three very good reasons to live the best life I can, with or without my hair. Those three reasons need their mama.

I took a small step on Thursday toward facing one of my greatest fears. In no way do I think those were the last tears I will shed about my silly (gigantic) head of hair, nor do I look forward to going through the next few months without it. But I did something really, really hard. And in a strange way, I came out feeling like I'd won a small victory.

P.S. In the Everything You Never Thought You'd Need For Cancer section of the store, I found these. And purchased them. And I've been pleasantly surprised to find that they work a little bit.

Now I Know

Friday, April 02, 2010

I AM EMERGING FROM THE fog of chemotherapy for a few minutes, just to let you know that I am still here. Chemo Day #1 went as well as it could have gone. It got off to a rough start with 3 different nurses trying 5 different times to start an IV, but after that it was uneventful, long, and slightly boring. As predicted, I have not felt well in the last few days. I am nauseous, but not throwing up. As long as we stay on top of the nausea medications, they seem to be doing their job of managing those particular symptoms. I am extremely tired, and I sleep a good deal of the time. I don't have any energy, but I trust that some of that will be restored in the next few days. Headaches come and go. Goliath was startled when he walked in and I was wearing a cool gel mask (helps with blood flow to ease headache pain). He said softly to Hubby, "Daddy, Mom looks like Zorro, only with a blue mask." I am supposed to be drinking a lot of fluid, but I'm having trouble getting it all down. I woke up this morning with that infamous metallic taste in my mouth—ick! A friend suggested hard candy, specifically Life Savers, to help with that, and it turns out that she was right. The three little cowboys seem to be doing fine. They

Allyson Hendrickson

are enjoying quality time with their dad and their tireless Nana! We know that the hardest days are still to come, and we so much appreciate your prayers for our family as we put our faith in the One who goes with us. "Be strong and courageous. Do not be terrified; do not be discouraged, for the Lord your God will be with you wherever you go." Joshua 1:9

Week 2 Recap

Friday, April 09, 2010

IT IS 4:42 A.M., AND I have been wide awake for almost an hour. This is just another way in which my body has betrayed me... it is very confused about our sleeping schedule. I am nearly to the end of Week 2 of my new Life o' Chemotherapy. Friends are sending me Facebook messages and kind e-mails wondering how things are going. I was trying to think of a good analogy for this and here's what I came up with: I feel like one of the poor little lizards that Little Middle loves to catch and keep as his "pets" in the summer months. Chemo has made me feel stuffed in a jar, with just enough holes cut in the top to get some air. Week 1 had me flat on the bottom of the jar—no stirring, just surviving. Week 2 has allowed me to move around a little bit. Every day I feel a little bit stronger and more "normal," although it does feel like someone keeps picking up my jar and shaking it to get a good look at what I might do next. Hopefully Week 3 will be even better and I can climb the rest of the way to the top, towards freedom. When we went to "chemo school" a few weeks ago, the nurse ran down an endless list of possible side effects. I was listening, but still holding out hope that most of those wouldn't apply to me. I'm not the typical interperitoneal chemotherapy patient, you know. I'm young, and other than the cancer that invades my body, I'm healthy. That's kind of a joke, ha ha. So now I know that the drugs are more powerful than the mind games I was playing. Nausea is at the top of the list! From the second day forward, I felt sick. Never actually throwing up is a big mark on the positive side, but the icky feeling…ugh. The good news is that I have 5 different medications that treat the nausea symptoms. I try not to think about what I would have felt like without those meds. Another big obstacle has been food. I have never had an issue with food—EVER—and all of a sudden, I can't eat. I don't even want to be close to food! Chemo changes the senses of taste and smell. I'm still navigating these waters to find out what works for me and what doesn't. The biggest disappointment has been my lack of taste for all things sweet. My family has enjoyed some of my favorite desserts while I hide in my room to avoid them. Sigh. You also hear about chemo patients feeling fatigued. I have discovered that there is a big difference between "tired" and "fatigued." Tasks that should be fairly simple—like drying my hair or sorting laundry—can easily become overwhelming. I am learning how to lower my expectations for myself and break my days up into sections, so that I can try to accomplish smaller things and still get the rest that I need. Of course, the last major thing I was concerned with was the possibility of hair loss. I was given this disheartening statistic at chemo school: 100% of Taxol patients lose their hair. 100%. The odds are stacked against me. Preparations have been made and many tears have been shed. The waiting is hard. Nonetheless, Hubby and I pray every day that God would single me out to be the first person in the history of oncology to keep their hair while undergoing treatment. It could happen. All of this sounds kind of pitiful. I hate to be a downer, so here are a few things that have happened this week that I have the sense to be thankful for: 1. After 8 days of being in the house, I drove myself and the boys to Bahama Bucks where we enjoyed the first shaved ice of the season. Baby chose Blue Bubblegum flavor, and his lips (and cheeks, and nose, and shirt…) were stained blue for two days. 2. I am in awe of the bluebonnets that have sprung up and the green, green grass and trees. His Creation is beautiful. 3. My family enjoyed dinner together, with all 5 of us sitting at the table. 4. I went to the park with my dad, my kids, and Abby dog. I watched my daddy organize all the neighborhood kids into a great game of soccer, and loved seeing my boys run and play in the sunshine. 5. I received the gift of a coffee table book filled with pictures from a family photo shoot we did before I started chemo. The book is beautiful, as are the hearts and the talent of the two friends who blessed me beyond words with it. He is still good. I said to the Lord, "You are my Lord; apart from You I have no good thing." Psalm 16:2

Broken Hallelujah

Wednesday, April 14, 2010

With my love and my sadness
I come before you, Lord.
My heart's in a thousand pieces,
Maybe even more.

The last few days have been filled with small joys and great sorrow. I was in the backyard on Sunday afternoon with Little Middle and Baby. Hubby had taken Goliath to Lowe's, giving the three of us a chance to play playdough on the picnic table without interruption. While we rolled out the pieces we needed to build The Longest Road Ever, I told the boys that Mommy is going to lose her hair because of the chemo medicine. Little Middle had a few tears and sniffles, and even more questions. "Why does the medicine do bad things to you, Mommy?" "Will you be sick again if you don't have any hair?" "Will you look like Poppy?" (That one made me laugh.) Baby listened intently, but finally got fed up. He put his little hand on his hip, looked at his brother, and said, "Little Middle, it is okay, because God is taking care of Mommy." Then he went back to building the playdough road.

Hubby and I had decided that we would do everything we could to prepare our sons for what is to come. After all, they are just as much a part of this family as we are, and they deserve to know what is going on. So after we enjoyed a takeout dinner and a little bit of classic Star Wars, I put on my wig (aka "pretend hair") and pulled out the hats/scarves we had purchased. We let the boys see how much the pretend hair looks like my real hair, and allowed them to try on some of my hats. Each hat has a name—there's the Swimming Pool hat, the Bank Robber hat, the Blue Bandana (which is actually a beautiful floral print scarf, but my kids like the word "bandana" because that is what cowboys wear), the Karate Kid hat. Little Middle and Baby had a great time modeling for us, and we were able to snap some pretty funny pictures. Goliath, on the other hand, did not enjoy our little family meeting at all. He kept a safe distance from me the entire time, and did not say much. As soon as he was able, he escaped to his room, and when Hubby went after him, he was laying on his bed crying. I took over (I felt a sense of entitlement—it's MY hair, after all!). But after I lay down next to him and wrapped him in my arms, I was lost. All I knew to do was to hug him and tell him that I love him, and that God loves him. We cried together for a long time, and it felt like he was comforting me just as much—maybe more—as I was comforting him. After a while, the tears stopped, and he whispered these words: "Why is this happening to us, Mom?" I swear I heard my own heart break.

I don't know, baby. I DON'T KNOW.

How could I doubt your goodness, your wisdom, your grace?

Oh Lord, hear my heart in this painful place.

On Monday, I got up early, and after dropping off my two older boys at school, I headed to a place where I love to be: preschool! I have the best class of 4-year-olds, and I have missed them terribly. I have been feeling pretty good this last week—good enough to go back to teaching, at least for a little while. I was tired after a few hours, and left around 11:30. But those sweet little friends were every bit as happy to see me as I was to see them…the smiles on their faces made every minute worth it!

On Monday and Tuesday evenings, I volunteered to be the parent on Sports Duty. I took Little Middle to his karate class and to soccer practice. My boy athlete amazes me…I love to watch him learn new skills and play. In spite of his quiet nature, he loves karate, and is quite good at it! I especially enjoyed watching him spar. He went four rounds, and won each time! On the soccer field, he is fast and swift. He listens carefully to his coaches, and tries hard to follow their instructions to a T. He swells my heart.

These seem like small things, but I have missed them so much! My life is being a wife and a mom. These four people I live with are everything to me. There is nothing I would not do to protect them and keep them from being hurt. It feels like my prayers are falling on deaf ears—is it really too much to ask that I am able to keep my hair? But this truth from my childhood still rings true: Jesus loves me, this I know. I will continue to trust and praise Him, even when all I can offer is a broken hallelujah.

When all that I can sing is a broken hallelujah When my only offering is shattered praise
   Still a song of adoration
   Will rise up from these ruins
   And I will worship You and give You thanks
   Even when my only praise is a broken hallelujah.

Housekeeping, Home Health, and Hair

Friday, April 23, 2010

Today is Day #3 of Chemo #2. As I write this, I am propped up in bed, sucking on a watermelon-flavored Jolly Rancher (darn that metallic taste!). Without a doubt, this round of chemo recovery is going more smoothly than the first. I know that there are many prayer warriors who have asked this specific thing for me, and I am humbled and very aware that God is answering those prayers. Thank you, friends. Chemo Day (Tuesday) was uneventful. It took one nurse one try to get an IV started. That alone was a vast improvement over last time! Hubby and Mom were with me the whole day. Three people in one small room for eight hours might seem a little claustrophobic, but there's no way I could make it through these treatment days without them! To pass the time, Hubby and Mom work on various professional and personal projects, and I write thank-you notes, read, and sleep when the Benadryl kicks in. I had a change in perspective toward the end of the day. The lady in the room next to me was obviously having a very difficult time. We could hear her vomiting every few minutes—difficult to listen to, excruciating to live through. The chemo nurse helped her as much as she could, but when the worst of it was over, she pulled up a chair to the lady's bedside and gave her this grim news: "At this point, there is no way to continue this course of chemotherapy for you." The conversation continued quietly, with the woman's husband asking what—if any—other options might be available. I was floored. I have been so wrapped up in feeling sad about my cancer and my chemo, that it hasn't really occurred to me to be truly thankful. What if I was the lady on the other side of that thin wall? What if Nurse Michelle had to say to me that chemo was no longer an option? Lord, forgive me for taking this awful, life-saving medicine for granted.

On Wednesday morning, Mom and I drove back down to Dallas for my Neulasta shot.

Neulasta is a must during chemotherapy! It boosts my white blood cell count and helps protect against infection, especially during these days when my immune system is compromised. The labs I had done last week were right on target, so I guess it's working. Also on Wednesday, I received a much-needed, much-appreciated gift. Precious friends from our Sunday School class are sharing their housekeeper with us! I was a little nervous when she dropped by earlier in the week to get a look at the house. I obviously have not been doing much (okay, any) cleaning. I showed her around and watched her carefully as she worked out some fancy housekeeping equation in her head. It had something to do with the number of bedrooms + the number of bathrooms– the pity she felt for me = how much she will charge. While she was figuring, Goliath charged in the front door, cheeks bright red and breathing hard from riding his bike. The next second, Little Middle and Baby ran through the back door, fresh off the trampoline. The air was filled with the smell of sweaty little boys. The tiny Latino housekeeper looked at them with an open mouth and said to me, "Ohhhh…you have three boys?" I nodded and introduced the stinky boys to her by name. She looked at them again and said (this time more to herself than to me), "TRES?!? Oy, Dios." Then she offered to knock 5 more dollars off the price of weekly housecleaning. She left my home that evening probably feeling grateful to Dios that she is not me, and I felt like I had won the lottery! I had an appointment with Dr. M before I left for the wedding last week. He asked a lot of questions about the first round of chemo: how I felt, how long it took for me to get "better," symptoms, etc. He was not too thrilled with my report that it took a good 7–8 days for me to be semi-functional. According to the good doctor, most patients need about half that time after a chemo treatment to begin to feel more like themselves. He attributed some of that listlessness and extreme fatigue to possible dehydration. So, in an effort to ward off dehydration this time around, he put in orders for a home health nurse to come out to my house and run fluids. Nurse Debbie came for the first time yesterday. After nearly 2 hours, all of the paperwork was filled out, and my Caretakers (Hubby and Mom) were trained in hooking up an IV line, operating the pump, proper sanitation procedures, saline and heparin injections, and even removing the needle from my arm. It was pretty fun last night, especially given my drugged-up state of mind, to watch Hubby act as my own personal nurse. He did a great job, though! I will do another 8-hour IV drip today, with the final one tomorrow.

About my hair…I wasn't sure I would be able to write about my hair on the blog. I can write about cancer, my family, my faith—but somehow, telling you about my hair makes me feel extremely vulnerable. But over the course of the last week, as I stood next to my best friend during her wedding, and danced with my husband, and survived another day of chemotherapy…I was reminded that there are literally thousands of people who are faithfully bringing my name before the Father every single day. Many of you are my friends and my family members, but there are MANY more who have never even met me…yet you continue to pray. That's not something I take lightly, so I

Allyson Hendrickson

want you to know everything—even the things that feel ultra-personal. Early last week, my hair began to fall out. After a couple of days and one traumatic shower, it was obvious that I would not be the first Taxol patient on the planet to keep her hair. So I made the heartbreaking decision to go ahead and take care of it before I went to Houston for Caroline's wedding. Mom and I went to Survivor Gals, and she held my hand and sang to me while the stylist shaved my head. I could feel the hair sliding off my head and the tears rolling down my cheeks, but I still felt a sense of disbelief—a "no-way-is-this-really-happening-to-me-right-now" feeling. I did not look at my bald head until late that night. I was safely locked in the bathroom, ready to wash my face, when I peered in the mirror. One glance was all it took to sink me to the floor and consume me with shoulder-shaking sobs. I don't know why it is that my hair seemed so important, or why losing it has been so devastating. I feel real grief over it! I also feel ridiculous and impatient with myself. I have a disease that could KILL me, and I have spent much more time and energy worrying and grieving over my hair than anything else.

It's been just a little more than a week since I lost my hair. In some ways, it seems MUCH longer. It's amazing what you can get used to if you simply have to. In all of the pre-hair-loss discussions, I had promised the boys that I would never go out in public without my "pretend hair." The last thing I want to do is make this more difficult for them! So when we go out, or when other people are around, I wear my pretend hair. But when it's just us at home, my head is covered by a hat, scarf, or turban. All three little cowboys seem to be adjusting just fine. Last night, after his shower, my precious Goliath came out of the bathroom wearing clean pj's and my black Bank Robber hat. He did not say one word about it, choosing instead to crawl up in bed with me and cuddle. No words were necessary.

Some days I look in the mirror and tell my reflection that yes, I can DO this. That I AM doing it! Other mornings, I look and all I see is a shell of the old Allyson. Some days are sunny and hope blazes through; other days are clouded over and doubt and depression linger like the smell of sickness. I hate those days. It is on those days that I remind myself that, sick or not sick, I am precious to God. "For you are a people holy to the Lord your God. The Lord your God has chosen you out of all the peoples on the face of the earth to be his people, his treasured possession." Deuteronomy 7:6

I am chosen. I am treasured. And with my God's help, I will beat this!

Snuggling with my Baby.

Hat time with Nana!

Love Lessons (Re)Learned

Monday, April 26, 2010

It is true that in several ways this round of chemo hasn't been as bad as the first. I have had less nausea, fewer headaches, and not as many days curled up in bed. In other ways, it has been more difficult. The fatigue I feel is extreme. It has been difficult to find the right balance of food for my system. And the emotional strain is more. So much more. I was surprised yesterday when I looked in the mirror and saw a sick person staring back at me. There was no trace of the old laughter, love, or life in my face. Instead, I saw baldness, weariness, and sadness. How did that happen so fast? How did cancer jump in and steal my joy when I wasn't looking? While I was studying my pitiful reflection and wondering what happened to ME, something even more surprising happened. My husband walked in behind me and told me I was beautiful. He kissed my bald head. He wrapped me up in his strong arms— those arms that are carrying the weight of the world right now— and held me close. He said over and over again that he loves me, and that cancer will never change that. This man promised nearly 12 years ago to love me, no matter what. He promised to give me the best of himself, in good times or in bad. He promised to help me and protect me, in sickness and in health. He is a man of his word. And you know what is really amazing? He tells me that he's a little bit glad we are facing this disease together, because cancer is teaching him what love really is. We were so young when we got married! We were fresh-faced and ready to take on the world. Sometimes, I take inventory of our life: house in the suburbs, SUV with a soccer ball rolling around in the backseat, 3 noisy little boys, 3 pets. Long gone are the days of sipping wine during a leisure Friday night dinner, or taking a whole weekend to watch the Rocky marathon on HBO. No doubt that he loved me then. But now…there's a whole different element to us. We never could have imagined that the fire we would walk through would be this hot. One thing's for sure, though: there is no one else I would want walking by my side. Babe, there are not words that would be adequate to express everything you are to me. How you manage to maneuver through each day and still be yourself is beyond me. I love the man that you always have been, but especially the man that you are right now. When I need you the most, you amaze me…over and over and over again. Thank you for taking out IV lines and dispensing medications. Thank you for working so hard and traveling when you have to, even though I know you dread it. Thank you for spending so much extra time with the boys and making them feel like all is right with the world because their daddy will take them fishing. Thank you for making me feel safe, and loved, and still pretty. Thank you for being who God made you to be: the perfect one for me. I love you.

This Sums It Up Nicely

Thursday, May 06, 2010

It goes without saying that cancer has turned my world upside down, but it felt like the final straw when I had to give up my morning coffee and exchange it for caffeine headaches and hot tea. I don't even like hot tea!

A few weeks ago, a long-time friend of our family sent me this delightful little gift:

I sip my hot pomegranate tea each morning out of this mug. I still miss my coffee, but I enjoy the feeling of satisfaction this disrespectful mug gives me. And let's be honest: the mug is right.

Blog Bulletin

Monday, May 10, 2010

Tomorrow, May 11, 3 Little Cowboys will go live for the first time!

I will give you a peek at a day in the life of a chemo patient by blogging from my chemo treatment room. Check back throughout the day for updates.

I'll meet you back here tomorrow!

Live Blogging Event: Chemo #3

Tuesday, May 11, 2010

Good morning! So many friends, family, and even praying strangers that I haven't had the pleasure of meeting yet check in here at 3LittleCowboys regularly to get updates on me and my family as we journey down the winding road of The Sickness. Many of you have asked me about my chemo treatments, so I thought it would be interesting (if not fun?) to give you a glimpse of a typical treatment day. I will update this post throughout the day as people come and go and things happen. Check back often, and when you do, scroll to the bottom of the post to read the latest! So, without further ado, here is my first live blogging event!

5:30 a.m. Alarm goes off. I drag myself out of bed and into the shower. Shower doesn't take long because I don't have any hair on my head to wash or hair on my legs to shave.

5:40 a.m. I feel better. I dress, go to the kitchen, turn on the coffee pot and empty the dishwasher.

5:50 a.m. I sit down with my computer and 1/2 cup of coffee in my favorite mug. I check my e-mail and post this verse as my Facebook status:

> No, in all these things we are more than conquerors through Him who loved us. For I am convinced that neither death nor life, neither angels nor demons, neither the present nor the future, nor any powers, neither height nor depth, nor anything else in all creation, will be able to separate us from the love of God that is in Christ Jesus our Lord. (Romans 8:37–39)

6:07 a.m. I put on makeup, fix my "hair," and start taking my morning pills.

6:30 a.m. I bring Hubby coffee and gently remind him that we need to leave in 25 minutes.

6:40 a.m. I toast an English muffin and finish packing up my stuff to take to the doctor's office.

6:44 a.m. Goliath is sleeping on an air mattress on the floor in our bedroom. I don't want to wake him up, but it sure is hard to make our bed in the dark!

6:46 a.m. I need to brush my teeth, but Hubby has locked me out of our bathroom while he is in the shower. Grrrrr.

6:50 a.m. I am ready. Hubby is not.

6:57 a.m. We rush out the door. We try to be gone on chemo mornings before the boys wake up at 7:00. We are supposed to be at chemo by 7:30.

7:00 a.m. We are driving down our street, and Hubby suddenly pulls over and jumps out of the car. We have a flat tire. REALLY?!?

7:02 a.m. We dash back through the house looking for keys to his truck. The boys are all up. Everyone needs a hug from Mom. We are now officially running late.

7:06 a.m. We forgot to get Sister's wedding invitations out of the crippled SUV. Mom and I are going to stuff them today during chemo to get them ready for mailing. We go back home again.

7:10 a.m. Finally on the road. We have to be there in 20 minutes. I really, really hate being late! Traffic is bad. We are thankful when we finally make it into the HOV lane, but Hubby gets mad when he sees that the guy driving the minivan behind us is the only occupant in the vehicle. He blows smoke out of his big truck onto Minivan Man.

7:45 a.m. We made it! I apologize to the nurses for being late, but they assure me it's no big deal. I can't tell if they mean it or if they just feel sorry for me.

7:55 a.m. Nurse Stephani gives us a few minutes to settle into our room. The only nice thing I have to say about chemo days is that, as an IP (interperitoneal) chemo patient, I have a private room. I don't know what I would do if I had to spend these hours in the "big" chemo room with other sick strangers. Stephani starts an IV. Today my best veins are on my right side, and the IV goes in my wrist. That makes it a little harder to type/write/etc. because I am right-handed, but it's OK. 2 bags of saline fluids are started through the IV drip.

8:08 a.m. Nurse Michelle brings me a cup of water. I can not figure out how to get the straw through the lid.

8:15 a.m. Hubby has to leave. He is going to work at a customer site for a few hours this morning. He kisses me goodbye and promises to be back as soon as possible. I am thankful that there is work for him to do.

8:22 a.m. Stefani came in to hook up the 2nd IV line to my IP port. Ouch. She starts another bag of saline through that line. All this fluid is supposed to expand my belly to make room for the chemo meds later in the day. I have to lay in a reclining position for a while.

8:52 a.m. Mom just got here. She reports that the boys got off to school and that Goliath was grouchy this morning. Sigh. She figured out how to get the straw into my water. Good thing, because I was getting thirsty and I hate drinking without a straw.

9:31 a.m. Nurse Karen came in to check on me. The saline bag attached to my port is finished. She disconnected it. Yay! Mom and I are listening to a new CD she has of kid's music. One song in particular is a perfect reminder for me today of God's sovereignty and love for me. Here are partial lyrics:

Where were you when I crafted you a language?
And where were you when I filled your mind with words?
So you could cry, so you could sing
Sprinkle names on everything
So you could laugh, tell a joke
Imagine towers wreathed with spokes
So you could live and die with dignity
And shake your fist with poetry
Imagining creation from the first.
Where were you?
When I laid the earth's foundations
Where were you when I set the stars in place?
And they all sang together
They all sang together up in space.
Allelu allelu alleluia
Allelu allelu alleluia.

9:58 a.m. My "friend" from the room next door just poked her head in to say hello. She is quite the Chatty Cathy, and is not always reassuring about what is coming next for me. Still, today is her last treatment, and I am happy for her. The lady in the room across the hall is on her 3rd phone call. She uses treatment days to catch up with her friends on her cell phone. I can hear everything she says—her grandson Braden has a sore throat that she hopes is not strep. Mom and I are about to get started on the wedding invitations.

10:25 a.m. Karen came in and started the Emend drip. Emend is an anti-nausea medication. I will also take it in a pill form at home tomorrow and Thursday.

10:50 a.m. Stephani started me on Zantac and Benadryl drips. We had better hurry up and finish the invitations before I fall asleep!

11:03 a.m. Zantac and Benadryl are done. Stephanie started the Aloxi (another nausea med) and the Decadron (steroid) drips. These are the last of the pre-meds before the actual chemo drugs get started in a little while. We are about halfway through with the invitations. I told Mom that I hope she doesn't die from licking all those envelopes, like Susan on Seinfeld.

11:18 a.m. IV pump is beeping. It does that sometimes when I move around or it just is in a bad mood. Nurse Stephani to the rescue! The last two pre-med bags are empty and she just brought in the Taxol bag. Taxol is the drug that goes through my IV port, and is responsible for my hair loss. I'm not a fan of Taxol. Stephani flushed my IV line with Heparin to make sure it is still working. It is. I can hear someone vomiting down the hall. Mom has an envelope-licking-induced headache. Hubby just called to report that he is meeting our good friend Jamie for lunch and offered to bring us Pei Wei. Yes!

11:34 a.m. Stephani came in with the lunch menu. Dr. M treats all of his chemo patients to lunch on treatment days. He's really a nice guy. I'm holding out for Pei Wei, though, so Mom went down to the vending machine and brought back peanut butter crackers and Skittles to tide me over until Hubby's return. The regular receptionist is out today because her daughter had a baby last night. The sub receptionist lacks people skills and wouldn't let Mom back in the office. She is not a favorite of ours!

12:09p.m. My brother is on the phone with our mother complaining about the length of this play-by-play post.

12:55 p.m. Hubby is back and Pei Wei is here! Orange peel chicken—yum!

1:03 p.m. Invitations are done! All 215 of them are stuffed, sealed, and set to be mailed out later this week. You're welcome, Seester.

1:22 p.m. Stephani says it's time to start the Cisplatin. This chemo drug goes directly into my abdomen through my port. It is responsible for the nausea and all the food upset that I've experienced. I'm not a fan of Cisplatin, either, but they tell me it's saving my life. I am taking out my contact lenses and getting ready to watch one of my favorite movies: Dirty Dancing. If you don't hear from me for a while, it's because I've fallen asleep. Thank you, Benadryl.

2:11 p.m. Stephani came in to answer questions and discuss important dates that are coming up. One thing to note is that I will have a CT scan 2 weeks from today. I am a nervous wreck about this scan...the one I had in January did not show the 2 tumors that were growing, so I've lost whatever confidence I had. Plus, the scan itself makes me sick. But Stephani assured me that the scan is important, and if it raises questions, Dr. M will not hesitate take action and order further tests. The lady across the hall is on the phone again discussing speed limits.

2:34 p.m. Taxol and Cisplatin are done! Stephani took the needle out of my port. There is still 1/2 a bag of saline flowing through the IV pump.

2:48 p.m. Stephani added Lasix (a diuretic) to my hydration. Johnny Castle and Baby are practicing lifts in the lake for their Sheldrake Hotel "Mambo Magic."

3:11 p.m. Hubby just left to go pick up the boys. We will all meet back up at home in a bit.

3:25 p.m. IV pump is beeping again. The hydration is empty! While we wait for a nurse, Mom and I are reading your precious blog comments and Facebook messages to each other. What an encouragement you are!

3:28 p.m. Michelle disconnected the IV and I am headed home!

4:39 p.m. We made it home and I am safely in my own bed. Hubby is on a work-related phone call and Mom/Nana just left with the boys to get some Baskin Robbins. All is well. I feel icky, but I am asking God to show mercy and favor during the coming days. This concludes today's live blogging event! I hope you've enjoyed following me today. Who knows? Maybe we'll do it again sometime. Thank you so much for caring and especially for praying. I continue to stand on my faith in the Almighty God and trust Him, quite literally, with my life. He is good, and He does good.

Halfway There

Saturday, May 15, 2010

It's the weekend. Weekends used to be such a sweet time around here—a time for sleeping late, big breakfasts, and taking it easy. Now that The Sickness is part of us, weekends blur together with all the other days of the week. This particular Saturday morning finds me back in bed (again), watching the clouds gather outside my window. They match my mood. I had not expected the treatment on Tuesday to be fun, but I anticipated it as an important milestone: I am now halfway done with chemo! The treatment schedule includes six sessions, the last of which will be on July 13. My thrill at being halfway done, however, has been shadowed this week by a slow recovery. The Caretakers (Mom and Hubby) and I now believe that chemo is at least somewhat cumulative…each treatment adds to the poison that is already lingering in my body and makes it harder and harder to bounce back. One major difficulty that I have experienced is severe and lingering leg pain. Last Friday morning, while I was at school, I received a call from Stephani that my lab work had come back with magnesium levels that were less than spectacular. I had to leave school, drive to Dallas, and sit through a 2-hour magnesium infusion. Granted, the mag did help with the leg pain, but by Wednesday it was back again. I called the office yesterday to report it, and by the end of the day yesterday I had been to the lab, had blood drawn, and had a bag of magnesium delivered to my home. I will do the 8-hour infusion today, along with regular saline hydration. I am told that this is not uncommon. It is the nature of the chemo beast to attack not just the bad cancer cells, but a lot of good things in the body as well...like magnesium and potassium levels. But to me, it's just one more thing in a long string of things to deal with.

I am tired of not feeling well. I am tired of seeing the worry and sadness in the eyes of the people who love me. I am tired of being tired. I am tired of missing out on LIFE. I told myself when this ordeal started that I would always look for the proverbial silver lining, even when it was really hard. This week feels darker than others, yet I still have joy. Here's how: *Yesterday my precious 4-year-olds graduated from preschool! It was very important to me that I be there, cancer or no cancer. So I got dressed, put on some makeup and my happiest face, and went to cheer them on. I got to shake hands with each little one, give them a Bible of their very own, and tell them I love them. I wouldn't have missed it for the world. (Big props to the Caretakers for not arguing with me about attending!) *Hulu.com has allowed me to enjoy the delight that is Glee with minimal commercial interruptions. Mom and I watched 3 episodes together last night. My friends tease me that my perfect life would be like one big musical where everyone breaks out into song regularly. Glee is that life, and it makes me happy! *My children. Those 3 boys fill our home and my heart with amazing joy! Yes, they are noisy, and yes, we have to remind them over and over again to PLEASE not bounce on Mommy's bed, but when Goliath brings me a cup of hot tea that he made, or when Little Middle climbs up for a hug, or when Baby pops his head in my bedroom and says "I wuv you," I remember that every minute of this fight—no matter how hard—is absolutely worth it. We are hard-pressed on every side, yet not crushed; we are perplexed, but not in despair; persecuted, but not forsaken; struck down, but not destroyed." 2 Corinthians 4:8–9

Anxious

Monday, May 24, 2010

IT'S A BIG WEEK IN my little cancer bubble. Now that I am half way through chemotherapy, I am scheduled to have a CT scan tomorrow. The scan, like those I've done before, takes pictures of my insides to see if there is any cancer growing. Unlike the ones before, however, tomorrow's test will answer our most important question: Is the chemo working? We don't really expect to see any cancer—after all, I just had all visible cancer surgically removed a few months ago. But before we can forge ahead, Dr. M has to know what's really going on inside.

To say that I am anxious about the scan would be an understatement. The last one I had was in January, when I had two tumors growing in my abdominal cavity. The images revealed elevated fluid levels, but no shadows of those tumors. My confidence in the technology significantly deflated at that time—and now this is what we are depending on to give an accurate picture of what's going on in my body? I am uncomfortable, to say the least.

But I have confidence in my doctor, and even greater confidence in my God. Even on that day in January, before I knew what was happening, He was with me. He was in the room with Hubby and me on February 17th when the devastating diagnosis brought our world to a screeching halt. He was with me on the first day of chemo, and He was there when my hair started to fall out. God saw my tears fall yesterday as I watched my three babies playing and wondered if I would live long enough to watch them grow to be men. He knows that I am scared, but that doesn't change the way He feels about me. And as for me? I don't understand why He does what He does, but I know without a doubt that He is good.

On Thursday, Hubby and I, along with my parents, will meet with Dr. M to get the test results and confirm the course of action for the next few months. I am so thankful for the prayers and petitions you are lifting up on my behalf; this week, would you join me in praying these things?

- minimal physical discomfort
- calmness of spirit, mind, and body
- crystal clear images that reveal exactly what needs to be seen
- positive results
- safe travel for my mom and dad

You are good, and what you do is good. (Psalm 119:68)

What Cancer Cannot Do

Thursday, June 03, 2010

CANCER IS LIMITED:

It can't cripple love,

It cannot corrode faith,

It cannot eat away peace,

It cannot destroy confidence, It cannot kill a friendship,
It cannot shut out memories, It cannot silence courage,
It cannot invade the soul,

It cannot reduce eternal life, If cannot quench the spirit,
It cannot lesson the power of the resurrection. Charles Swindoll, The Finishing Touch

The Weight of Suffering

Saturday, June 05, 2010

FOR FOUR DAYS NOW, I have hidden in the cocoon that is our bedroom, hunkered down beneath the raging storm of chemotherapy. I am sick. I am exhausted. The Caretakers tell me that at times I am hilarious. At one point yesterday, the cloud of nausea lifted enough that I actually felt hungry. I went to the kitchen and toasted an English muffin. Mom came in and asked what I was doing. I replied, "I'm just fixing myself a mid-morning snack." She laughed hard, because it was in fact 1:15 p.m. and morning had come and gone without me even knowing it!

I have been more out of it during this round of chemo than any other. I'm at the point now where if I could, I just might want to throw in the towel and forget the whole thing. Forget the nauseous, could-get-sick-at-any-minute feeling. Forget the ever-present disgusting taste in the back of my throat. Forget the leg pain that lingers and the endless supply of pharmaceuticals that are lined up in our bathroom cabinet. Forget the look on my Baby's face when he spotted the IV needle in my arm. Forget the bills pouring in and the incessant questions, poking, and prodding by strangers. FORGET CANCER.

But somewhere in the recesses of my clouded mind, a soft voice persists. It tells me to press on. It tells me that yes, I am definitely swimming in the deep now…deeper water than I've ever been in before. But that I am still safe. Just a little while longer. I am not treading water for nothing. That my name is engraved on the palm of His hand (Isaiah 49:16), and that those mighty hands can be trusted, even in the midst of my suffering.

> The burden of suffering seems a tombstone hung about our necks, while in reality it is only the weight which is necessary to keep down the diver while he is hunting for pearls.
>
> —Jean Paul Richter

When Life Hands You Lemons…

Wednesday, June 16, 2010

I RECEIVED A GIFT YESTERDAY from some friends. Neither the gift nor the givers are what you might expect, but both are extraordinarily precious to me.

You see, the friends who gave me this gift are small—not much taller than 4 feet. And they are five years old and have not yet been to kindergarten. But their hearts are HUGE. Their gift was in a simple envelope addressed to "Ms. Allyson." The envelope contained a card that had this picture on the front:

Inside the card, there were 3 carefully written names. And money.

It took me a minute to put it together, but when I began to understand what exactly the gift was, I was stunned. My small friends had a lemonade stand. FOR ME.

The emotion I felt was overwhelming. I literally sank to the floor and wept. My little friends watched me carefully…I think they were worried that I was sad! I hugged and kissed them, assuring them that I was VERY happy with their gift to me.

D said, "Ms. Allyson, you can give the lemonade money to the doctor and he can give you a lot of medicine so you can get well." Oh. My. Goodness.

According to the moms (also my friends) of these 3 delights, the kids have been wanting to do "something nice" for me since they found out that I am sick months ago. Together they came up with the idea for a lemonade stand and worked very hard to make it successful!

And successful it was! Trust me when I tell you that a lot of generous people must have been very thirsty on that hot summer morning. Apparently, an e-mail went out to many friends who showed up to help and/or buy lemonade. Lots of little ones took turns holding signs and manning the shop.

Every time I look at these pictures, I feel like my heart could explode with gratitude. And pride. And love. And JESUS. Because what these pictures really show is love in its sweetest, simplest form.

Thank you, friends. Life has handed me lemons, but you made lemonade for me. I am blessed beyond belief.

Opposites

Thursday, July 01, 2010

Tonight during dinner Little Middle and I were playing the Opposites Game. It's a favorite around here: I say "up," he says "down." I say "white," he says "black." You get the picture.

After a few rounds, I asked him, "How are you and me opposites of each other?"

He said, "Well, you're big and I'm little." Right.

"You're a girl and I'm a boy." Uh huh.

"You're a grown-up and I'm a kid." Yes!

"I have hair and you don't." Ouch.

All the bravery and good humor in the world can't change the truth. And sometimes, the truth really hurts.

An End in Sight?

Friday, July 16, 2010

THE ONE THING I AM wishing for this morning is that there is an end in sight. An end to the treatment, an end to the sickness that keeps me hidden in my darkened bedroom. An end to this terrible illness that has taken over our lives.

Tuesday was Chemo #6, the last one in a rigid protocol of treatments that many women are unable to complete. Knowing this, I feel slightly proud of myself and tremendously thankful that I was able to see it through to the end. The stamina it took to finish did not come from me, but from the power of God that was granted to me through intercessory prayer.

The effects of #6, however, are by far the worst I've dealt with. I am SICK. I have zero energy or motivation to try anything. When the boys come in to see me, it is as if I am divided into two moms: the best part of me wants to snuggle with them and reassure them; the worst (and most honest, hidden) part of me wants them to just go away because I simply CAN'T DO IT. I am unable and unfit to be the mother they need me to be right now. If you know anything of my heart and my affections for those 3 little cowboys, you are able to recognize the enormity of that admission.

The only thing that truly seems to make these days bearable is to sleep my way through them. I am on a constant cycle of sleep-inducing, nausea-reducing drugs. I slept my way through most of yesterday, and plan to do the same today (and tomorrow...and maybe even the next day). I have always thought that it would be the easy way out, and have hesitated in previous chemo rounds to sleep around the clock. This time I honestly feel like I might not survive if I have to be aware of how badly I really feel.

This pity party is enhanced by something we learned during chemotherapy on Tuesday. The term "maintenance chemo" has been tossed around in front of us previously, and I finally got up the nerve to ask Nurse Stephani about it. Of course, the final decision will be made after I have a PET scan and meet with Dr. M next month, but Stephani gently communicated that it is a very real, and highly likely, possibility that I am not done with chemo. To be fair, maintenance chemo will not be anything like what I am currently going through. It would most likely be a Taxol cocktail, administered 1 day a week for 3 weeks, then 1 week off before the next round. Two things that prick my heart: 1) A new Taxol protocol means that my hair will not grow back anytime soon, and 2) I just want to be DONE. As long as my name is still on a blue folder (for patients actively receiving treatment) in Dr. M's office, I am in a sad place.

"Relent, O Lord! How long will it be? Have compassion on your servants..." Psalm 90:13

From the beginning, I have tried to make it a point to look for things to be thankful for. That seems much harder to do during these dark days, but here are a few things that are happening RIGHT NOW that make my heart smile:

1. My mother is sitting next to my chair, reading over my shoulder. She has been here through every treatment,

taking care of my household and my boys while I am unable to. I am thankful.
2. I can hear the sounds of my three boys playing and laughing together in the other room. I am thankful.
3. My husband is in his man-cave/office working on a project for a job that we have been unsure he would be able to keep at times. I am thankful for steady work and God's protection of his job.
4. Even when I don't feel like it, the knowledge that is rooted deep in my heart tells me that my God is faithful and is in control of all things. I am deeply thankful.

What Next?

Monday, July 26, 2010

NOW THAT CHEMOTHERAPY IS DONE, the big question is: What next? Well…tomorrow, July 27, I will have a PET scan done in Dallas. Dr. M has heard my concerns and agreed that every other scan on my new imaging schedule (every 3 months) will be a PET. The technology is more sophisticated, the results are more reliable, and the testing is much easier on me than the conventional CT scan. My insurance company is unhappy, but that's OK. Sorry, Aetna. Then, on August 2, we meet with Dr. M. He will give us the results of the PET scan and make his recommendations for what to do next. We fully expect the scan to be clear—if it's not, then what good has all this chemo done?—but the expectations for the future are uncertain. Of course, I am asking God for healing, as I have done every day for the last five months. I believe that God can remove all traces of this disease from my body, and keep it away. But if there's one thing I've learned through all of this, it is that God can still show Himself through me—regardless of my circumstances—if I will simply step aside and allow Him to work. More of Him, less of me. Will you pray with me?

Today I Learned...

Monday, August 02, 2010

- that last week's PET scan was clear.
- that "clear" doesn't necessarily mean "cancer-free."
- that I will have to do maintenance chemotherapy for six months.
- that maintenance chemo is designed to be a cancer preventative and buy me some time.
- that without the maintenance chemo, I could expect the cancer to return in less than a year.
- that there is a blood test I can do that can determine my sweet sister's genetic predisposition to my disease.
- that it is definitely not OK to take 12 Tylenol in one day.
- that my port will stay in until sometime next year.
- that after a cancer patient has one reocurrence, the chances of another reocurrence skyrocket.
- that a lunchtime margarita doesn't heal, but it helps a little bit.
- that it is very scary to have a best-in-his-field doctor look you in the eye and say that you are a random case and he

simply can't explain why things are happening the way they are.
- that my husband and my parents are extraordinary.
- that faith is being sure of what we hope for and certain of what we do not see. (Hebrews 11:1)

This Hurts

Friday, August 06, 2010

THERE HAVE BEEN A FEW times in my life that I have felt such acute emotional pain and fear that I knew I would never be the same. Like watching a dear friend sit with her 3-year-old daughter at her side during her mother's funeral, and when another precious friend wept over the coffin of her father. When we dialed 911 after a 10-month-old Goliath had a seizure in his crib…when I endured a hysterectomy and had to dismiss the dream of having the 4th baby that I desperately wanted and would have loved so much…when my brother walked through a seemingly endless, horribly dark time, and I could do nothing but love him and feel helpless…and a few others that are too personal—and sometimes still too hurtful—to share here. Last Monday was one of those times. Yes, the PET scan was clear. And I am grateful. What I am still trying to absorb is Dr. M's revelation that there are almost certainly cancer cells—however minuscule—somewhere in my body, just waiting to multiply and form new tumors. Cells have to be a certain size to be detectable by radiology. Just because we can't see them doesn't mean they aren't there. In my case, they probably are. One of the reasons I love and trust Dr. M is that he is forthcoming with vital information. His job is not a pleasant one; I honestly don't know how he does it day in and day out. My cancer is pretty much guaranteed to come back. We asked him about a timeline for that, and while it was obvious he didn't care for the question, he gave a straightforward answer. If I participate in maintenance chemotherapy, I can have maybe 2 years of "normal" living. If I don't, new tumors can grow in 9–10 months. That news stopped me dead in my tracks. In 2 years, my Baby will be just six years old. He will be learning to ride a bike without training wheels. Little Middle will be building those mega Lego sets instead of the medium-size ones he loves now. Goliath will be reading encyclopedias for fun and asking crazy questions about stuff we've never heard of. In 2 years, they will still need their mom. There is still a lot I want to do. I want to have a cabin in the mountains where my Hubby and I can go to be alone. I want to take my kids back to Disney. I want to learn how to decorate cakes. I want to read new books. I want to teach until kids make fun of me for being old. I want to do a Beth Moore Bible study and not skip around on the homework. I want to volunteer and make a difference to someone, somewhere. I want to go to New York with my friends and to Europe with my sister and my mom. There is so much living left to do! And that is why I feel so much sadness and fear. Because I know now, with greater clarity than ever before, that my life and my dreams are threatened by The Sickness. Not only will it come back once…it will keep coming back, over and over again. I will never again feel safe from the clutches of cancer. I will always wonder if it is there, secretly lurking and growing. I will always be aware that at this very moment, I might be dying. Our Bible Study lesson (does anyone call it Sunday School anymore?) this morning was about hypocrisy…why non-believers are so turned off by the Christian community as a whole. We all agreed that it is because our lips and our life don't match up a lot of the time. In other words, we say one thing and do another. I don't want that to be me! I want to be genuine, so that's why I can't say that I'm not scared. My world was rocked last week. I am looking hard for God, but for the first time I feel mad at Him. At the same time, though, I know that the medical timeline is not the same as the one God has for me. I believe there is still plenty of space for a miracle to happen. There doesn't have to be another recurrence. I am overwhelmed by what I know could happen, but my faith is firm. I will be purposeful in trying to follow the instruction from 2 Timothy 3:14: "But don't let it faze you. Stick with what you learned and believe…" (The Message) Lord, this hurts. I need you to be the strength that I just don't have right now. I believe that you are still good and your plan for me is perfect. Please help me to be real and honest for those who are watching, but most of all, for you. Dry my tears and turn my sorrow into joy. You are more than enough for me.

New Normal

Thursday, August 26, 2010

THE NON-CANCER BLOGGING EVENT HAS come to an abrupt end. I am typing this from the chemo room at Dr. M's office. I am hooked up to an IV, and Taxol is being pumped into my veins. I am surrounded by five other women, all older than me, most bald like me. Maintenance chemotherapy has begun. Yesterday, Mom, Hubby, and I met with one of the oncology nurses for a chemo teaching session. None of the information was necessarily new or startling. The new protocol utilizes Taxol (a chemo drug that I was on previously) and Avastin (an antibody) to prevent recurring cancer. We know that the reality is that in my case, the cancer will almost certainly return—the maintenance protocol is hopefully just slowing it down some. I will come in every Thursday for chemo—3 weeks on, one week off, for the next six months. Those four weeks together are considered to be one "round." After the third round, I will have a CT scan done; after the sixth round I will meet with my doctor and re-evaluate. I am told that the side effects should be much less than the hell I endured with the "big" chemotherapy. Most patients experience a day or two of fatigue after a treatment; nausea and muscle and

Three Little Cowboys

bone aches should be significantly less, if I even experience them at all. I will have to go to the lab every week on the day before chemo and have a Neulasta injection after the third week in every round. Neither of these routines is new. All in all, I guess I should be thankful. Compared to where I've been and what I've done, this should be a piece of cake, right? But here's my hangup: I don't want to compare the next six months to the last six months. I don't want to drive to Dallas every single week to sit in this room with these other sick people and know in my heart that I am one of them. More than anything, I don't want to explain to my sons what I have to do and wonder how to answer their questions. I want cancer to GO AWAY. I want to go back to the life I had before The Sickness. I want to be freed from the cloud of doubt and fear that seems to follow me wherever I go. After the meeting yesterday, Hubby and I hugged my mom and she headed home to Houston. We got in our car, and my emotional dam unleashed a waterfall of tears. I am exhausted from this. I have fought hard, and I worry that I just don't have what it takes to keep fighting. The last few weeks have been as close to normal as I have felt in a long, long time, and I have loved being able to do the things I used to do before I got sick. I am so MAD that I have to give that up again and replace it with this new normal! I am reading a little book by Anne Graham Lotz called *Why?*. In it, she says this: "There is more to life than being healthy, than being happy, than being problem free, than being comfortable, than feeling good, than getting what we want, than being healed. There is more to life even than living! And the 'more to life' is the development of our faith to the extent that our very lives display His glory!" Just a few weeks ago, my friend Becky (who is also the boys' music teacher at school) sang in the worship service at church. The chorus of her song had these lyrics: I'm satisfied I'm satisfied I've been cared for so faithfully. But Lord, hear my plea And may it be That you're satisfied with me. I will not stop asking for healing. I will not stop believing that God is in the miracle business and that I can live a long, happy life. But even over that, I want to make those song lyrics my own prayer: May it be, sweet Jesus, that I draw power from you that I don't have on my own, so that every breath I take points right back to you. I want to dig deeper and look harder to find satisfaction and contentment in what you've given me, so that you shine.

> In this you greatly rejoice, though now for a little while you may have had to suffer grief in all kinds of trials. These have come so that your faith—of greater worth than gold, which perishes even though refined by fire—may be proved genuine and may result in praise, glory and honor when Jesus Christ is revealed. (1 Peter 1:6–7)

I have a long way to go before I can honestly rejoice in my circumstances, but I will work on it! In the meantime, I will drive to Dallas every week and I will sit in this room with these other sick women. I will trust my God, love my family, and believe that there is a plan in place for me…and that it is very, very good.

About the Hair

Friday, August 27, 2010

I WOKE UP AT 4:04 this morning and the first thing that popped into my head was that I should probably say something about my hair on the blog. I couldn't go back to sleep, so here I am.

It is still very hard for me to talk about my hair, but I am committed to being an open book. Here goes: It's no secret that chemotherapy took my hair. I have been bald since April. Around the house I usually wear a hat or a scarf, but the deal I made with my little cowboys was that I would always wear my "pretend hair" when we go out. Always. And I have stuck to that promise (except for that one unfortunate day when we were on the way to the swimming pool and I had to make a desperate run into Walgreens, so I sacrificed my dignity and went in wearing my swimsuit under a coverup and my straw pool hat).

Chemo took the hair on my head a long time ago. What you may not know is that more recently, it took my eyebrows and my eyelashes. To be exact, it stole my eyebrow. One. The only thing dorkier than walking around with no eyebrows is walking around with only one. I grieved the loss of that rarely-thought-about hair on my face almost as much as I mourned the hair on my head. At least I can cover up my head; losing my eyebrow and eyelashes made me look sick.

In the six weeks since Chemo #6, I have noticed that my hair is trying its best to make a comeback. Hubby says my head looks like a baby's—the hair is very fine and sticks straight up. I also shaved my legs this week for the first time in I don't know when! There is still no sign of the eyebrow growing back, but if you look at my eyes really closely (mostly from a side view) you might see the teeny tiny little eyelashes that are growing. They are still way too small to put mascara on, though. I tried yesterday, and all that got me was a makeup MESS all over my face.

So what next? Taxol is the drug responsible for my hair loss, and it is the drug that I will continue to take during maintenance chemo. Yes, it will be a much smaller dose than what I had before, but still! I asked Nurse Michelle about it, and she said that I can expect continued hair growth, but the Taxol will slow it down considerably. Also, any new hair that grows will probably be thin and brittle. Great.

Mom and I visited Survivor Gals this week to see about getting a replacement wig. Even if I wasn't going back on Taxol, it will still be a long time before my hair grows enough for me to be comfortable to go without my pretend hair. Mom and our wig expert Kathy encouraged me to try a new style. Change just is not my friend. In the end, I ordered new hair that is exactly like my old hair…but I changed the color slightly. If you see me in a few weeks parading around with my blonder color and chunkier highlights, please tell me you love my hair. Even if you don't. It will make me feel good if you make it believable. (Wink.)

Also, if you see me, don't look too closely at my one eyebrow. I learned some makeup tricks, but Lord knows I'm no Bobbi Brown. Mom bought me this button at SG. Right now it is pinned to the outside of my makeup bag. I think I will use a Sharpie marker and cross out the "S" on the end of "eyebrows." Then I will wear it, maybe not proudly, but at least with a blossoming sense of humor.

Bits and Pieces

Saturday, September 18, 2010

- I have had a great coffee week! First this…and then I discovered this:

YUM.

- The calendar says we are just days away from the official start of fall, but you wouldn't know it if you came to Dallas. Any day that has a heat index of less than 100 degrees is a good day. Come on, autumn!
- Fall may not quite be in the air yet, but change certainly is. My Hubby took a leap of faith and a good opportunity and began a new job this past week. He resigned from his position of five years and went to work for a Fortune 300 company that specializes in metal products as a senior network engineer. The biggest change? He is going to an office every day as a regular 8-to-5er. The best part is that the new job requires only about 10% travel…significantly less than what he has been doing. I am so proud of him, and so very thankful for God's provision.

- This is my bye week for chemotherapy. I was very much looking forward to a "normal" week with nothing medical going on, but it was not to be. The instant I woke up on Tuesday I knew that something wasn't right. I was dizzy and lightheaded, and my heart was beating fast and hard. My amazing friends stepped up to help with the boys, and I laid low most of the day. When it wasn't better on Wednesday, my chemo nurse helped me make an appointment with a general practitioner that Dr. M trusts. Turns out that what I was experiencing were anxiety attacks. Although I don't necessarily feel anxious (or any more so than usual), the GP explained it like this: You can only stretch a rubber band so far, or put so much tension on it before it snaps. Thanks to cancer and chemo, my body can't handle life as well as it used to. The anxiety attacks are my body's way of saying, "Whoa—this is too much!" I am trying to listen and take it easy, and with the help of a new medication, I have felt better the last few days. Still, I am a little bitter that there is another medical thing to worry about. Sigh.
- I keep finding the little cowboys perched here: and Gus hanging out here:
- Two dear friends had to say goodbye to their beloved pets this week. My heart aches for them in their losses, and I have snuggled my Abby dog just a little tighter in the last few days.
- Baby and I baked chocolate chip cookies together as an after-school treat for his brothers. As we put them in the oven, he said to me, "Mommy, this has been a good cookie experience."
- One of the most bothersome side effects of my chemo is peripheral neuropathy. I have it in my feet, and I want it to GO AWAY.

- I bought razors this week for the first time in six months. It has become necessary to shave my legs every few days.
- My brother is getting married this afternoon. There will be a whole other post about that later, but for now…I see his joy and it fills my heart.
- My family drank 4 1/2 gallons of milk last week. I think it would be cheaper and more efficient for us to have a cow in our backyard.
- I have really, really amazing and caring friends.
- My sister was in a car accident this week. She was hit by an ice cream truck. She is completely fine, but her husband's Mercedes Benz is definitely NOT. I'm not a bad sister, but I giggle every time I think about that ice cream truck. And they didn't even offer her a fudgesicle!

Teal Toes

Tuesday, September 21, 2010

WITH OVARIAN CANCER IS 60.

Did you know that September is Ovarian Cancer Awareness Month? To celebrate, I got a pedicure today:

A few facts about ovarian cancer:

- Ovarian cancer is often referred to as the "silent killer," as the symptoms can easily be missed or mistaken for other ailments.
- There is no reliable screening method for detecting ovarian cancer, nor is there any real test designed to catch it before it spreads.
- The median age for women diagnosed
- Ovarian cancer is the 9th most common cancer, accounting for about 3% of cancers among women.
- Ovarian cancer is the 5th leading cause of cancer death among women in the United States.

- About 21,880 new cases of ovarian cancer will be diagnosed this year in the U.S., and about 13,850 women will die from the disease. I will not live in fear. I will not let cancer define me or steal my identity. I will continue to fight. I have teal toes!

Good News

Friday, September 24, 2010

SEVERAL WEEKS AGO, I GAVE a blood sample for the BRAC analysis test. In addition to all the "regular" cancer stuff, I have carried the weight of worry that people I love will be at a higher risk for cancer because of me. The BRAC analysis checks for gene mutations that would indicate the possibility of that happening. Yesterday during chemo, Nurse Michelle pulled me aside and said that they had received the test results. She handed me a folder, and in the middle of long paragraphs of medical mush, these words jumped off the page at me: NO MUTATION DETECTED. The tests were negative. My Seester, my cousins, even my children are not at any greater risk for cancer than the average person walking down the street. Thank you, Lord. Michelle handed me a tissue for the tears that were falling, and all I could manage to say was, "I love them so much." And I do. Now, just a touch of funny. Now that I have to go to chemo all by my lonesome during the maintenance phase, my mom and I have a plan worked out. I keep my phone close by my side and text her during the treatment. That way, she knows everything that is going on and I don't feel so lonely. Here is the series of texts that we exchanged yesterday: Me: Oh Lord. Just got here. 2 old couples in the waiting room discussing the beauty of Mackinaw Island in the summer. Mom: Don't make eye contact. Me: In sick room. One bald head, 2 sleepers, 1 Bible reader with 4 bottles of water. Dr. M just came by and kissed my cheek. Me: Houston, we have snoring. Mom: Make up a song about the chemo room. "All I want is a room somewhere..." Me: New addition who looks alarmingly like (someone we know), only taller. Mom: How many can fit in the room?????? Me: 6. It's always full. Me: Old lady a few chairs down has had a voice change b/c of chemo. She sounds like a man with a cold. Mom: Oh no. The dreaded voice change. Me: Sick lady is watching a how-to video on her computer about insurance—with no ear muffs! (I once mixed up the terms "ear phones" with "ear muffs" due to chemo brain. My mother still is laughing about it.) Mom: She should know muffs are a must in the chemo room. I can't make this stuff up.

Chemo Is Not Loverly

Monday, September 27, 2010

Picture Audrey Hepburn singing these words…my twist on a classic favorite:

All I want is a place somewhere far away from this chemo chair where women have no hair

Oh, chemo is not loverly.

The nurse says be careful what you eat
I say I still can not feel my feet
Off week is such a treat
Oh, chemo is not loverly.

Not so loverly sittin'
abso-bloomin'-lutely still
I want to cry when it comes in view just over the hill.

Three Little Cowboys

Old ladies staring straight at me
Talking over my misery
Oh, where is Stephani?
No, chemo is not loverly.
Loverly, loverly, loverly—
No, chemo is not loverly.

Ultimate Chemo Brain

Sunday, October 03, 2010

MY SISTER AND HER MISTER were in town this weekend for the Texas-OU game. I don't want to discuss the game itself, or the fact that they ate a deep-fried PopTart at the fair, so I will entertain you with a true story of chemo brain instead. I fixed Waikiki Meatballs for dinner last night (thanks, Dee!) and there was enough to feed my hungry Seester when they got back from the fairgrounds. I fixed her a plate piled high with meatballs, rice, steamed sugar snap peas, and bread. I handed it to her, she set it down on the table and excused herself to the bathroom. While she was gone, I cleared the table of all remaining dishes,—including her untouched dinner—brushed all food into the trash can, and loaded the dishwasher. When Jenny came back to the kitchen, she said, "Hey, who took my food?" And you know what I did? I helped her look for it. Oh, yes, I did. Thank you, chemotherapy, for destroying my brain cells but giving my family a reason to laugh at me.

I Want to Say…

Thursday, October 07, 2010

I wrote a new post earlier today while I was in the chemo room. I went back and read it, and realized it did not make a bit of sense. Crazy drugs and crazy people will do that to you. The crazies will also crush your ability to put together coherent thoughts, stand up straight for any length of time, or tolerate any noise/chaos/changes without wanting to pull your hair out (if you had any to pull). I have a lot to say, but I don't feel like I am able to get it down well enough or fast enough to justify telling it. Would you put up with one more bullet point list? Thanks. I want to say:

- That maintenance chemo is harder than regular "big" chemo in a lot of ways. At the top of the list: Going every single week. Thursday used to be my favorite day of the week, and now it is my least favorite. Even The Office can't make Thursdays OK for me anymore.
- After suffering debilitating leg pain, days-long headaches, and extreme fatigue, I spoke up and told Nurse Stephani that maintenance chemo was not at all like "drinking

water," as I was told it would be. She agreed that something is amiss in the way my body is responding to the treatment; I have an appointment scheduled with Dr. M on October 18th to discuss what could possibly be wrong and what we should do to fix it.

- I talked with each of my boys and now have their blessing to walk around the house with my head uncovered. Goliath told me that I "look like Uncle Phil, only a girl" with my "new" hair growing in.
- Gus the dog is able to get into more trouble now that he's tall enough to reach more stuff. His cousin Moose refers to him as "that giant puppy."
- I really want to take the boys to the state fair, but I don't know if we can make that happen this year.
- I like to mark in my books when I read. I just finished a book that is so marked up, I don't know if it will even be helpful when I go back to look for something specific. This book tore me up in a good way, and it took me forever to read it because I kept having to stop and absorb the information and apply it to my situation. It is entitled to its own post later on.
- We are being blessed by friends bringing dinner to our house twice a week while I am doing maintenance chemo. A lot of those friends don't seem to think that their gift of food is adequate. Hear me loud and clear, you cooking pals 'o mine: There are days (like today!) when your aluminum dishes full of warm goodness make me stand in the kitchen and cry tears of gratitude. You are doing for my family what I can not do, and that is HUGE to me.
- Earlier this week, city workers came out to repair the sidewalk in front of our house. Baby and I went out and sat on the grass and watched the workers mix, pour, and smooth concrete for the new sidewalk. Little boys love big

trucks, and he was a terrific mix of wonder and questions. I love that littlest man, and I loved making that memory with him. He reminds me why I must press on and keep giving everything I have.

- The Neulasta injection I receive every month costs $4,150.00. For ONE SHOT. Let that sink in.
- Insurance is so necessary, but is also such a pain in the rear.
- I love my job. I appreciate it even more now for the sense of normalcy it brings to my life.
- I still have two kids who need Halloween costumes.
- It is hard for me to answer when people ask me "How are you feeling?." I want to be honest, but I don't want to sound like I'm complaining.
- I really wish my sister and brother lived close to me, but I'm thankful for my very cool brother-in-law who does.
- My family is getting used to Hubby being at work all day. We are all adjusting to the new schedule, and we all really like it (especially the part where he comes home)!
- I've had a few lay-it-all-on-the-table talks with God lately. I've been very honest in telling Him that I am weary, and I just don't think I have what it takes to keep on going. I cry. I whine. I beg for Him to make it all go away. He tells me that He is nearby (Psalm 14:17), that I am safe (Psalm 91:1–2), that He has good plans for me (Jeremiah 29:11), and that there should still be joy in the midst of my troubles (James 1:2–3).
- A couple of friends put on a Pampered Chef show a few weeks ago from which all proceeds were to be donated to Team Allyson. I don't know what kind of funds a typical show nets, but it seems like everyone I know bought something! I am so grateful, and so humbled. Thank you, friends.

Hopeful

Tuesday, October 19, 2010

I MET WITH MY ONCOLOGIST yesterday. The appointment was not routine, rather, I requested the meeting in order to discuss the difficulties I have been having with maintenance chemotherapy. A bit of background: When I began maintenance chemo in August, I was told that it would be no big deal in comparison with the IP chemo I had just completed. I was assured that I could resume my regular activities and that I would feel much like my old self. The nurse told me then that the maintenance chemo would be "just like drinking water." Well, someone apparently poisoned the water hole. The maintenance has been horrible. I have experienced many of the same symptoms that I had with the regular IP chemo: debilitating leg pain, prolonged headaches, and EXTREME fatigue, to name a few. The big difference is that with IP chemo, I could plan to be sick for a few days, but I knew I would gradually feel better before it came around again. On the maintenance regimen, I am always either going to chemo or recovering from having been there. It is a constant cycle of misery and trying hard to get ahead. Even worse, my precious family is paying a very high price. I have been unable to do much of what

I normally would. My Hubby is trying to take over for me in a lot of ways, but he is exhausted. I am doing minimal mothering, and the little cowboys deserve better. So I said that to Dr. M. I told him that the quality of life that I have with the maintenance protocol is unacceptable to me and my family. I told him that I needed a change. I was worried that he might try to assure me that everything is fine, so I was greatly relieved when I described my symptoms to him and he said, "None of these things should be happening!" Good—I thought I was going crazy. We spent quite a while hashing out the details of a new chemo plan. In the end, it looked like this: I will not be receiving Taxol at all anymore. The once-a-week Taxol IV has been replaced with a once-a-day-Cytoxan pill (When I googled Cytoxan, one of the search results was "types of medicine for cats with breast cancer." Yikes!). The Cytoxan is another chemo drug—not as preferred as Taxol—but well-tolerated and effective. I will continue to receive Avastin as an antibody every other week and participate in the clinical study for that drug. The schedule remains the same: I will have a CT scan at the end of this cycle (mid-November), and another scan at the end of the sixth cycle (February-ish). At that time, if no new cancer shows up, I will be released from therapy and we will continue to monitor with scans and physical exams. In addition to working out the chemotherapy mess, I also felt ready—sort of—to ask some hard questions. Up until now, we have dealt with whatever issue was at hand and pushed all of the looking-into-the-future things to the side. As my body and my treatment have changed, however, so has my thinking. As much as I wish it could be different, my reality is that my body is affected by a life-threatening illness. I very much want for Dr. M to tell me that without a doubt, I will live to be a very old woman. I want to hear that I will raise my little boys to be fine men. That I will sit in the front row at their high school graduations, that I will take them to college, and after I leave them in a dorm room somewhere, that I will go home and bake cookies for the care packages that I will send them. I want him to say that I will dance at their weddings and that their wives will be the daughters I never had. I want him to say that there will be plenty of time for Hubby and me to travel together, and to build our dream house with a huge porch where we will sip coffee in our rocking chairs when we are very old (but still very much in love). So I just asked him: Best guess… what does my future look like? Deep breath. Almost certainly, the cancer will return. Hopefully it will be a few years, during which time I will live like I want to live instead of living according to what cancer dictates. When it does come back, it will most likely redevelop in the pelvic region, and everything I've done this year will need to be done again. Will cancer kill me? Maybe, maybe not. Dr. M is noncommittal, although we got a big lecture about the power of positive thinking. All in all, the news and the steps taken have left me cautiously optimistic. I have been so sick for so long that I almost expect the next thing, whatever it is, to be bad. Today my weary body and my discouraged heart feel ready. I am ready to try again, and encouraged to start putting one foot in front of the other. The journey is l-o-n-g, and the steps are so small. At the same time, my God is SO BIG. Even in my days of despair, He has been faithful and excessive in the ways that He shows His love for me. "I will be glad and rejoice in your love, for you saw my affliction and knew the anguish of my soul. You have not handed me over to the enemy but have set my feet in a spacious place." Psalm 31:7–8 I am trusting You, Lord, as we take these next small steps together. Give me the will to keep up the good fight and to keep pointing back to You. Help me to be the best wife and mom that I can be to my guys. Thank you for walking with me and flooding the path with Your light when I can't see where to go or what to do. I will continue to hold tightly to Your hand and follow Your lead. Amen.

Plan B

Tuesday, November 09, 2010

It's been a ho-hum sort of week—and it's only Tuesday. Some of my blah-ness comes from the fact that my eyelashes are falling out again. I've been watching them with suspicion for several days, but yesterday morning when I was putting on makeup I realized there weren't even enough there to justify mascara. I called my mom at 6:30 a.m. crying.

Now, I know that in the grand scheme of things, eyelashes don't matter. Hair won't get me to heaven. My husband won't judge the temperature of our relationship on whether or not I can flutter my eyelashes at him. The boys won't remember that Mommy's makeup looked different from other mommies. But to me, in the here and now, it matters. It suddenly seemed to matter even more after I questioned my chemo nurse about it, and she told me that there is a very real possibility that I could re-lose the hair on my head as well.

I recently read Plan B by Pete Wilson. A friend gave it to me and wrote inside the book that it was "a good read, probably one you could've written." BD, I'm sure you didn't mean for this book to tear me apart, but that's pretty much what happened. It's

Allyson Hendrickson

been a long time since a book has affected me to the degree that this one did. And I think it got to me because the premise of the whole book is this: What do you do when God doesn't show up for you in the way you thought He would? That question is one I've wrestled with for quite a while now. I had lots of dreams and plans once upon a time. Those plans might have looked mundane and boring to some people, but for the most part, I've always known what I wanted from life. It was simple: I wanted to fall in love, get married, raise a family, and live happily ever after. Yes, I went to college, and yes, there are days that I think wistfully of that framed diploma gathering dust in a box in our garage. Some days I think I would rather run an office than a carpool, or I would like to make money instead of cookies. But my four guys remind me that I'm living my dream, and even on the hard days, I know I wouldn't trade it for anything. In the summer of 2007, though, my little world came to a screeching halt with a cancer diagnosis. It had never occurred to me that

I could become Wife and Mommy and then get sick. Since then, and especially this year, I have had to abandon my perfect Plan A for my life and accept Plan B. Plan B means that instead of giving my family homecooked meals every night, I am ordering more than my fair share of pizza. It means that some other kid's parent gets to share a new experience with my son because I can't go on his field trip. Plan B means that my Goliath frets like a little old man when he is away from me because he is fearful that something will happen and I won't come back. Under Plan B, my husband digs through a basket of wrinkled laundry to find clean clothes. I hate Plan B. If I didn't feel like the cloud of cancer was hovering over me so closely, I might find it humorous that God allowed this to happen to me. Really, God? Me, of all people? The girl who despises change and upset in the order of things? "Your dreams may not be happening, and things aren't turning out the way you expected, but that doesn't mean your life is spinning out of control. It just means you're not in control." (Wilson) Ouch.

Three Little Cowboys

No doubt about it: I am definitely not in control here. I have spent much of the last 9 months asking God for a way out, begging Him for relief. I couldn't count the number of times I have said, "I just want my life back." Ironic, huh? I have walked with Christ for most of my life, but when we came to this, THE thing, I misstepped. I allowed fear and anger and uncertainty to creep in too close, and I begged God to give me what wasn't mine to begin with. I gave my life to Him a long time ago. I promised my husband on our wedding day that I would do my best to love him in sickness and in health—why would I do less for my God? This season of maintenance chemotherapy is hard. I fully expected that it would be much easier, both physically and emotionally, because—hey! I survived chemotherapy! The reality is far removed from my expectations. It still feels like chemo: I am tired, I'm taking LOTS of meds, I'm losing hair. The difference is that before, life was spinning around me, and now it is trying to sweep me along with it. A lot of days I feel like such a fake! On the outside, everything appears to be fine, but on the inside, I'm barely holding it together. What I know in my head doesn't match up with what I feel in my heart. One of my favorite quotes comes from Andy Stanley: "Every day we have this choice to make. Am I going to define God by interpreting my circumstances or am I going to simply trust that God is who he says he is?" My Plan B isn't at all what I expected, and certainly not what I wanted. But I think maybe I'm making it harder than it has to be by over-thinking. I might not ever know why God allowed this suffering. I'm not sure why it seems that He is silent at times when I need Him the most. Maybe it's time, though, for me to pull it together. "We're called to be faithful to God even when it seems he hasn't been faithful to us. We're called to love him even when we feel abandoned. We're called to look for him even in the midst of the darkness. We're called to worship him even though our tears." (Wilson) When darkness veils His lovely face, I rest on His unchanging grace. In every high and stormy gale, my anchor holds within the veil. His oath, His covenant, His blood, support me in the whelming flood. When all around my soul gives way, He then is all my hope and stay. I choose to continue to look deeper and love more, trusting Him through my Plan B.

This and That

Wednesday, December 01, 2010

I know there hasn't been much activity on the blog lately, but that's really because there hasn't been much to say. Cancer, along with its many sorrows and joys, is still with me. The new maintenance regimen is much better than before, but it is still chemotherapy. It's difficult. I am having a CT scan next Tuesday, and a follow-up meeting with Dr. M on Thursday. We anticipate that all will be clear, as expected, and he will recommend marching forward with what I'm already doing. Still, there is much anxiety as the day approaches. I would appreciate your prayers. Now, how about a little of this and a bit of that to catch up?

- Little Middle lost three teeth in four days. The Tooth Fairy is going broke. And he came home from school today with the announcement that another one is loose!
- I upgraded some of our Christmas decor this year. I figured after 12 years of marriage, we deserve a new tree skirt. Thank you, Hobby Lobby, for your over-the-top after-Thanksgiving sales!

- Speaking of Christmas decorations, Hubby and Goliath hung lights outside. We want to do outside lights every year, but it doesn't always get done. Ahem. Anyway, while they were working, I heard maniacal laughter from the backyard. Turns out that Little Middle climbed up on the roof and JUMPED OFF onto the trampoline. Be still, my heart.
- Baby's favorite indoor "decoration" is the Little People nativity set. He is constantly rearranging the animals and the characters, and pushing the angel down so she will "sing." He loves to sing along to Away in the Manger, and I cracked up when I heard his sweet voice sing "the little Bo Jesus laid down his sweet head." I mentioned that the right lyrics are "little Lord Jesus," and he said, "Hmmm. I always thought it was Bo Jesus." He keeps on singing it that way.
- Goliath is going to be Penguin #7 in the school Christmas play. It reminds me of this.
- I was totally blessed by two groups of MOPS moms from my church who adopted me as their "service project." One group took three baskets of our laundry to the laundromat, and the other group went to the grocery store for me. I literally wept when I saw the full refrigerator and the baskets of neatly folded clothes.
- Christmas came early for Hubby this year. He is the proud owner of his first new car since 1998. Believe me, he deserves it.
- I am on a personal mission to seek out joy this holiday season. It isn't coming as naturally to me as it usually does, so I am being very intentional about looking for it.
- While we were in Houston, my brother invited my boys over to his house for Nephew Camp. It might be the greatest thing that's ever happened to them—they are

still talking about it! Baby now wants to get a Christmas tree to use in his room for a nightlight, because "that's what Uncle Phil let us have."

- I could probably construct a small temporary shelter with the lint I pulled out of my dryer today.
- Gus the dog is no longer my friend. He ATE the blue cover that goes over the trampoline springs, for crying out loud! What's worse, he doesn't much care what I think of him. He only has eyes for Hubby.
- Princess Puppy Love has stiff joints now that the weather is cold. Watching her struggle to get up and down (and I don't mean because she's plump) makes it easier to forgive finding her hairs on my new black sweater.
- I am not a fan of the new hair growing on my head. It is curly and it is the color of ugly dirt. The good news is that my eyelashes are finally growing back.
- When Hubby changed jobs back in September, we paid to COBRA our health insurance for about six weeks, until his new benefits kicked in. They were quick to take our money, but have yet to pay out one single claim that my doctor's office has made. What's more, we haven't been able to do much about it because we didn't get our ID cards until two weeks after COBRA was up. This has been so frustrating!
- Every single room in my house has at least a few silly bandz scattered around the floor.
- When I got up this morning, I got my glasses off my nightstand. It wasn't until I turned on the lights in the kitchen that I realized I was wearing my sunglasses.
- Goliath did a family tree project for social studies. I enjoyed helping him put together the information and telling him stories about the memories I have of my great-grandparents.

- One of my favorite things my husband does for me is to get the coffee pot ready every night. Each morning when I get up, there is already fresh coffee waiting!
- I bought something on Cyber Monday for the first time ever.

Scared

Thursday, December 09, 2010

IT IS AN AWFUL FEELING to wake up in the morning and think, "Today is the day I will find out if I have cancer in my body."

That is how my day began. Before I even opened my eyes this morning, my heart was pounding, my stomach was sinking, and I was begging God for favor. Maybe I should back up a bit… On Tuesday, I went to the hospital for my every-three-months-regularly-scheduled scan. This was a CT scan, much more difficult and not as detailed as a PET scan. When I got to the hospital and checked in, the technician took me and my sweet mom to a back waiting room and delivered 1 1/2 hours worth of barium sulfate. I had to drink a certain amount every 10 minutes. Let's just say that the more I drank, the faster the 10 minute mark kept coming! Before I even had time to rejoice that the cocktail was gone, the tech returned and whisked me back to what is really a closet with a chair in it. She started an IV, and then we went to the imaging room.

I've lost count of the number of times I've laid on that table, trying to follow the instructions from the automated machine: "Breathe in. Hold your breath." Whrrrrr. "Release your breath."

Whrrrrr. Up, down, in, out. If I open my eyes, when the table moves me out of the machine, I can see what I'm sure is supposed to be a peaceful scene on the ceiling—a flowing brook surrounded by towering trees. I much prefer to close my eyes, but then all I can see are the faces of my boys. Desperate terror was what I felt on Tuesday. I think I might have tried to jump off that table and run away, except that 1) I was trapped in the imaging tunnel, and 2) I had a needle in my arm that attached me to an IV pole. So instead, I did the only thing I knew to do: I recited Scripture. A scripture, to be exact: Isaiah 26:3. "You will keep me in perfect peace, whose mind is stayed on you, because I trust in you." (paraphrases mine) Over and over again.

The scan takes less than 10 minutes, but it seemed so much longer than that. Finally, it was done and I was free to go. I collected my things and my mother and practically ran for the parking lot. Once we were safely in the car, I lost it. I simply could not contain the anxiety and fear any longer.

I don't know why I feel so terrified every single time I have to go there. Besides the obvious, I mean. I think it's natural to feel scared. The threat is very real. But after all this time, why do I start to hyperventilate when the hospital comes in sight? Why do my hands shake when I enter the office? Why do I still cry? I'm not nearly as brave as I want to be, or as good as I should be. I feel like if I were, then 2 Timothy 1:7 would not resonate with me like it does: "For God has not given us a spirit of fear, but a spirit of power, of love, and of self-discipline."

Mom, Baby, and I passed the waiting hours of Wednesday doing a little Christmas shopping while the big boys were at school. After school, there were spelling words to practice, friends to play with, and iCarly to watch. I'm pretty sure I've seen every episode of iCarly that there is. We went to bed early, and that brings us back to this morning. "Today is the day I will find out if I have cancer in my body."

As it turns out, the scan was clear. The emotions I felt with that news were a mixed bag: Relief, fear, joy, sorrow. Of course it was good news! It was exactly what I, along with so many of you, have prayed for. In the back of my mind, though, I can still feel the fear creeping in. This clear scan is just a reprieve...a temporary sigh of relief. The Sickness will be back, unless God overrules medicine (and He absolutely could choose to do that!).

I explained it to a close friend this afternoon this way: I feel like Eeyore, who always moved around with a dark cloud hovering over his head. No matter where he went or what he did, that cloud stayed with him. That's me. The cloud of cancer follows me everywhere. Just because it's not raining right now doesn't mean it isn't there or that I am not acutely aware of it. It permeates everything I think and do. It threatens to open up and pour down on me at any time. And do you want to know the truth? I am scared of it.

I hate that I'm scared. I want to be brave. My boys make me want to be brave. Whether or not my time with them is cut short, I desperately want them to remember that I trusted my Lord with all that I had. I want them to know that I faced the Sickness, if not cheerfully, than certainly with a welcoming spirit for the challenge. I want them to know that they were worth fighting for, and that the strength that I had to fight came from above.

Tonight I cooked one of their favorite dinners and we celebrated the good news with root beer floats. Watching them enjoy their desserts, I breathed a prayer of thanks that there is "no evidence of recurrent or metastatic disease." I asked God to help me slow down and be present in the here and now, and most of all, to help me get a handle on that spirit of power, love, and self-discipline. If God is for me, who can be against me?

Confessions

Tuesday, February 01, 2011

OLD MAN WINTER BLEW INTO our city last night with a vengeance, and it seems he is settling in for a few days. I have some excited little cowboys who are not going to school today. It's going to be a Netflix-watching, pajama-wearing kind of day.

And I have to confess that it won't be the first day that I've stayed in my pjs recently. I've had a rough go of it lately. It started on my last treatment day, when the woman in the chair next to me cried the whole time. It was her first chemo treatment, and she was scared. Part of me wanted to comfort her, but most of me was annoyed and angry—angry that she had to be there, angry that I had to be there, and angry at cancer in general. That treatment room is a terrible place. Cutesy ribbons and bows on the IV poles and cheery green plants on a desk can not disguise the reality of what goes on there. It's awful, and I hate it.

The side effects of last week's treatment were tough. They always are, but for some reason I had a more difficult time bouncing back. My emotional state is directly related, to a degree, to my physical pain. The more my body hurts, the more my heart hurts. Tuesdays are treatment days. I typically go pretty early in the morning, and I am back home by lunch time. I like to stop off at Schlotzsky's on my way home and grab lunch, sort of like a reward for myself for enduring the morning. My order is always the same: a small original sandwich, hold the lettuce, onion, and tomato. I get home, change into my pajamas, pop the first of several pain pills, and eat my sandwich. Then I put my best game face on, deal with it, and wait to feel better.

Only this time, Wednesday morning came and I did nothing. I didn't shower or change clothes. I didn't put on makeup. I didn't dig deep and look for the silver lining. I'm not even sure I brushed my teeth. I just let myself be sad. I looked for the closest pool of self-pity and jumped in. I watched kid TV with Baby during the day, and when it came time for church that evening, I did not make the boys go. It was just too much effort. Good mom, right?

Then it was Thursday. I had to do something very hard that brought to light some tough issues. I've said it before, and I'll say it again here: I am not the only one affected by The Sickness. My suffering is not solitary; the sorrow isn't isolated. On that particular day, it simply felt like more than I could bear.

On Friday night, my family chose from these three options for dinner: blueberry Eggos, chocolate chip Eggos, and cinnamon microwave pancakes. Again, the mundane everyday task of preparing a meal required more than I had to give.

I am facing another scan within the next couple of weeks, followed by a meeting with Dr. M. That meeting will determine what we do next. I asked my chemo nurse, and she said he more than likely will want me to continue with the maintenance chemo, in spite of its "uncomfortable" side effects. The reasons are solid: theoretically, the longer I suppress cancer cells with the chemo, the longer it will be before they can grow again. Makes sense.

But the anxiety and depression I feel knowing what's coming is ridiculous. Nearly one year after the start of Chapter 2, I still find it hard to believe that this will be the rest of my life. When I started this journey, I said that I did not want to lose myself and be identified by The Sickness. But more and more, I am afraid that is exactly what has happened. Pretty much everything I do (or don't do—i.e. cooking dinner!) is determined by how strong or sick I feel. I don't make plans without checking to see when my next treatment day will be. I don't laugh like I used to, or even cry like I used to. Not too long ago, I watched Steel Magnolias with my Bible Study sisters, and I didn't shed a tear when Shelby died. Not one. I was stone-faced when M'Lynn lost it in the cemetery. And I can't remember for certain, but I don't think I even laughed when Clairee offered up Ouiser as a sacrifice for her friend.

I am reading a book right now titled The Gift of an Ordinary Day by Katrina Kenison. The author is a mother of two sons, and the book is her memoir. In reading, I have captured a glimpse of what I want more than anything: plain old, ordinary days. Mornings that allow me to sleep as late as I want to instead of my wake-up time being dictated by last night's medication. Afternoons that are open for game-playing or park-going or just plain lazing around with my cowboys. Evenings that invite us to share a home-cooked meal on the back patio and count the airplanes that fly by or wonder about the rooster that we can hear through our neighbor's fence. Days that are blank squares on my calendar instead of doctor appointments. Days that don't involve pills or IVs. Days that I can look in the mirror and like what I see. Normal. Is that really too much to ask for?

On This Day...

Thursday, February 17, 2011

ONE YEAR AGO TODAY, I sat in stunned silence as my oncologist told me that there were new tumors growing in my body.

The year that has passed since February 17, 2010 has been harder than I could have ever imagined it could be. Not one single day has gone by that I have not lived and breathed the reality of cancer. I have been sicker than I ever thought possible. I have had to rely on my friends and family to care for me, and even worse, to care for my children. I've had to try to explain things to my sons that no child should ever have to even think about, let alone live with. I've listened to my husband cry in the middle of the night when he thought I was asleep. I've been poked, cut, prodded, and tested, and I've swallowed hundreds of pills. I've lost my hair. I've lost my dignity. I've lost my confidence.

Today, in a twist of irony, I had another appointment with Dr. M. I was going to find out the results of the CT scan I had on Tuesday and hear his advice on how to proceed with treatment. After several heart-stopping moments where I strained to hear his conversation with Nurse Michelle in the hallway, he entered the exam room and pronounced that no new tumors showed up on the scan. A great deal of back-and-forth ensued. I will spare you the details, but the bottom line is this: I will continue with the cytoxan/Avastin maintenance regimen for a few more months. At the end of that time, I will go for another scan and if all remains unchanged, I will be declared to be in remission and this leg of the cancer journey will be over.

You'd think that with the end in sight, I'd be thrilled, right? Actually, I am terrified. The news on my latest scan is good, no doubt about it. But to me, it's not a sigh of relief…it's just a delay of the inevitable. I've been told more than once that the cancer will surely invade my body again. Just because it isn't there now doesn't mean it isn't coming.

Dr. M was prepared to release me from treatment today. He saw things through different lenses than I do, however. He looks at me and sees a challenge, a science experiment, a few dollar signs, and maybe an opportunity. I look in the mirror and see a wife, a daughter, a sister, a friend, and a mother. The whole time he talked to me (or sometimes over me) today, all I could see in my mind's eye were my 3 little cowboys. Their faces were so clear, in fact, that I did something a lot of people might think is ridiculous: I chose to continue chemo. I couldn't picture myself tucking my boys into bed at night, knowing that I could have done more to prevent The Sickness from recurring. I've come this far…what's a few more months?

So I will press on. I will do every treatment I can within the time frame I've been given. Cancer is a terrible disease. I hate those abnormal silent cells with everything I have. And February 17th? I don't care for it much, either. But next year, I will be able to look back and remember that this is the day I chose to finish strong.

After the appointment, my mom and I had lunch together. There's nothing worse than crying in a restaurant with people all around you laughing and enjoying their lunches. I am just so sad. Even good scan results feel like a burden to carry. I am well aware that this sounds like a woe-is-me, glass-half-empty kind of narrative. I don't mean it that way at all. In fact, just in the few hours since I saw the doctor, I hugged two friends, laughed with my boys, kissed my husband, talked to my sister, and snuggled my dog. I am blessed beyond measure. It's just that I am at sort of a breaking point with The Sickness…it seems to be controlling me more than I am controlling it.

The mug said it all.

Barbara

Monday, February 21, 2011

Almost thirty years ago, my parents moved our (then) family of four to Oak Ridge, a little suburb just north of Houston. The doors on the moving van had barely shut when we set out on the hunt for a new church home. We found that home at Oak Ridge Baptist Church—back then, it was known as "that big white church by the freeway." We hadn't been there very long when our family first got to know, and then to love, the Wolfe family.

Joe and Barbara and their sons Jody and Jamie were a typical American family in a lot of ways. Joe was a CPA who looked for any excuse to go fishing, Barbara taught school and took care of her family. They were atypical in a few ways, too. Joe suffered from polio as a child, and the effects of that followed him into adulthood, making it more and more difficult to walk.

Jamie had muscular dystrophy. As the years went by, the muscles in his body atrophied until finally he was wheelchair-bound.

You might think that life dealt this precious family a particularly unfair hand. Not one of them would have agreed with you. The love they had for each other and for God was unwavering. They approached life with enthusiasm and lots of laughter. Their faith got them through the darker days, and they made sure that God got full credit and glory in all things, good or bad. I watched them carefully through the years, especially Barbara. I couldn't have known then that I, too, would be the only girl in a house full of boys. She poured everything she had into her family and her church. I know she worked harder than I can even imagine, but no one that I know ever once heard her complain.

I grew up and moved away from my family and my church. My parents moved to the other side of Houston just a few months later. It's hard to keep in touch with people you don't see often, but we loved those Christmas letters Barb and Joe sent out! They were just as funny as being with them in person. I finished school, got married, and Hubby and I started our life together. As a young wife, Barb often came to mind as a role model for the kind of wife I wanted to be for my husband. The thought of her always made me smile.

Then tragedy struck for our friend. In just a few years' time, Barbara lost her husband and both of her sons. Three lives...three loves...three funerals. Then, the unthinkable. She was diagnosed with breast cancer, and later, ovarian cancer. Cancer seemed to those of us on the outside to be the greatest injustice, just adding insult to injury for someone who deserved it the least.

Barb fought hard. She endured multiple chemotherapy protocols. She lost her hair, grew it back, and lost it again. She continued to teach a women's Sunday School class. She continued to encourage and uplift other people, even though her suffering must have been great. I know she did, because one of those people was me.

Barbara's last scan showed tumors growing all over her body. She moved in with her parents, and was placed under hospice care within weeks. On Valentine's Day, God showed mercy and called her home. I wish I could have caught just a glimpse of her three able-bodied boys running to meet her! What a perfect day for a perfect homecoming!

Allyson Hendrickson

The last time I saw Barbara was at my brother's wedding in September. She sat in an aisle seat during the ceremony, and several of their wedding pictures have her in the background, smiling like witnessing Phil and Chelsea's love and vows was the best thing that had ever happened to her. She gave me a big hug that day and reminded me to keep on fighting the good fight. She told me that even cancer was no match for the power that I have through Christ. Cancer took Barb's earthly life, but whatever she is experiencing now is nothing to be mourned. Indeed, He has turned her mourning into dancing!

The summer that I was about the same age that my Goliath is now, Barbara was my VBS teacher. During that week of VBS, she challenged us to memorize Psalm 100. I met that challenge, and all these years later, that Scripture passage is still hidden deep in my heart.

Shout for joy to the Lord, all the earth. Worship the Lord with gladness; come before Him with joyful songs. Know that the Lord is God. It is He who has made us, and we are his. We are his people, and the sheep of his pasture. Enter into his gates with thanksgiving and into his courts with praise; give thanks to him and praise his name. For the Lord is good and his love endures forever; his faithfulness continues through all generations.

That, my friends, is quite a legacy. To be not just a teacher, but a doer of the Word…to make lifelong impacts on people…to believe He is good even when it doesn't seem like it, and to proclaim His faithfulness to anyone who will listen…that is who Barbara was. And it's who I long to be.

Well done, good and faithful servant. Well done. Allyson, Phil, and Barbara—August 2010

Hair Update

Thursday, March 10, 2011

It's been a while since I posted an update on my hair. Most of ya'll are too polite to ask about it, but the subject still comes up every now and then. So, here's what inquiring minds want to know: My hair is growing. In fact, I got it cut a few weeks back. I didn't cut it because it has grown to an unmanageable length, though. Don't get too excited! I cut it because it will grow faster and better if I do some upkeep on it, or so I am told. What I secretly am hoping for is that there will be magic in those scissors, and it will begin to grow in a completely new way. What's coming in now is a weird texture (curly) and a weird color (mud). I much prefer my old texture (straight, at least with the help of a flat iron) and my old color (salon-blonde). That's what my "pretend" hair is, and that's what I will wear until…well, until I say otherwise. The curly mud grows on, though, all crazy-like—so much so that it must be restrained these days. I have to wear a grippy headband-type thing to hold it back before I smush it all up inside the pretend hair. Wig-wearing was easier when I was completely bald!

I wish I could say that looking in the mirror is easier these days, but that wouldn't be exactly true. Besides the mop o' mess, I am annoyed at the pasty white color of my skin. I am disgusted by the weight I lost last year and have managed to put back on (The Sickness and I will share the blame on this one). I have HAD IT! with the little zit that keeps showing up on my chin, regardless of how often I wash my face. I'm not 14 anymore, for crying out loud!

For as long as I can remember caring, I have always wanted to. Have better hair…lose weight…apply makeup like an expert…have clear skin…update my wardrobe—you can fill in the blank with almost anything that equates with prettiness. I don't feel much more comfortable in my body as a grown woman than I did in the awkward-for-everyone adolescent stage.

Understandable? Maybe. Sinful? Probably. Truthful? Absolutely.

The Sickness has forced my hand in a lot of areas, but this is a big one for me. When Goliath was a baby, I used to recite this Bible verse to him (we had fun hand motions and everything!):

"I will praise you, O Lord, for I am fearfully and wonderfully made. Your works are wonderful, and my soul knows it full well." Psalm 139:14

Now, if I could be so easily convinced that God took perfect care to weave my son together, what makes me think He would just toss together a few ingredients and hope for the best when it came to me? And if I could so readily and easily praise Him for the three miracles that are Goliath, Little Middle, and Baby, why would I neglect to praise Him for the miracle that I am?

Any good 12-step program will tell you that the first step to recovery is admitting that you have a problem. I have a problem with my self-image. The next steps in my "recovery" can be found in the pages of my Bible, where it says that I am special and loved…cancer, curls, and all.

Do's and Don'ts for the Chemo Room

Tuesday, April 05, 2011

IN HONOR OF MY LAST day in the chemo room (!!!), I have put together a little list of do's and don'ts for basic etiquette. I tell the little cowboys all the time that manners matter…even in the chemo room. Here's what and what not to do.

1. DO mind your own business. We might have to share nurses, but my cancer is mine and your cancer is yours.
2. DO NOT ask me every time you see me if I've tried the peppermint-flavored water. Maybe I don't like peppermint. Or maybe I don't like water. Probably I'm running out of polite responses.
3. DO wear a nose strip if it keeps you from snoring while you nap.
4. DO NOT talk about nose hair. I do not want to hear about whether you have it or not, nor do I care to know whether blowing your nose is easier during allergy season if said nose hair has begun to grow back.

5. DO keep private information private. Just like sex, any conversation about bodily fluids and/or functions easily lends itself to a TMI label.
6. DO NOT offer to share your neck pillow or blanket with me. Ick.
7. DO NOT ask me about the specifics of my case. Chances are that I hate being here, and having to rehash the depressing details with a stranger only makes me hate it more.
8. DO cover your head. Chemotherapy is a beast, and we all know it. There is no need to flaunt what it has stolen from you, thereby reminding the rest of us what we have also lost.
9. DO NOT, under any circumstances, wear pajamas, a housecoat, your slippers, or a crown to the chemo room. No way can you keep your dignity if you do.
10. DO wear a bra. Please.
11. DO NOT say things like "These pole covers are so cute!" or "That was easy, wasn't it?" Nothing in the chemo room is cute or easy to deal with.
12. DO be very careful what you eat in the chemo room. Because Mexican food and chemotherapy don't mix.

Peace and Quiet

Saturday, June 11, 2011

It's Saturday night. My little cowboys are in West Texas starting their summer off right with their grandparents. Hubby is watching the UFC fight at his brother's house. Abby Dog and I shared a Schlotzsky's sandwich and now we are catching up on my recorded DVR shows and enjoying the peace and quiet.

I deserve some peace and quiet, if you don't mind my saying so. We bought a new house and moved. Preschool ended and I watched my Baby graduate. I kept on dragging Goliath and Little Middle out of bed and to school every day, long after every other school district in Texas was done. I had a less-than-enjoyable doctor visit (I am fine.). Finally—FINALLY—Summer 2011 is here! I usually am not a fan of summer. It's way too hot and there is a little too much quality time with the kids. But this year, I am more than ready.

The last day of school was tough. Because of our move, the boys will attend a different elementary school next year. I have done everything possible to get them excited: We visited the school book fair and bought—what else?—Star Wars books. We took a tour of the campus and met the counselor and the principal. We admired the playground. But I know that none of those things make it easy for my sons to leave behind their friends and favorite teachers. There were tears in all of our eyes when we walked out of the doors of their school for the last time.

We celebrated the end of school by heading straight to the pool. The first swim of the season was great! It's already 100+ degrees here. You know what they say about Texas…we have four seasons here: Almost Summer, Summer, Still Summer, and Christmas. Anyway, Baby was triumphant at the pool when I showed him that he is finally tall enough to touch the pool bottom in the lazy river, and that he is tall enough to go down one of the big slides. Victory! Now if we can just get him swimming confidently like his brothers…

We love, love, LOVE our new house. It is nearly twice as big as our old one. Each of the boys has their own bedroom, and they are really enjoying having their own space. I have a huge bathtub, a kitchen with two ceiling fans and more than enough cabinet space, and a laundry room that is an actual room. That hasn't endeared me more to the laundry chore, but it makes it a little easier to keep up! We have nice neighbors and fruit trees in the backyard. Our own little piece of paradise…aaahhh. Of course, no experience in this family is complete without some sort of mishap. We had lived here almost three weeks when our washing machine went berserk and we had a flood. The water in the laundry room was deep enough to cover the top of my foot when I was standing in it. Even worse, the Gain-smelling river ran straight into the hall where we have wood floors. I ran around town like a crazy person before I finally landed at Home Depot, where I rented a wet-vac and made friends with a sympathetic old man with chewing tobacco in his back pocket. With a little help from my good friend Momma Wolg, I managed to suck up the water, but not before it damaged the flooring. The silver lining: My feet smelled nice and felt super-soft from all that sloshing around.

Three Little Cowboys

Things have been pretty quiet here in CancerLand. Back in the spring, I went to M.D. Anderson in Houston. MDA has been on my radar for a while, but I haven't felt well enough to make the trip for quite some time. My reason for finally going was two-fold: One, I wanted/needed to get a second opinion about "what's next?" and two, MDA is renowned for their clinical trials and experimental drugs to treat cancer. Having been assured that cancer will forever be a threat, I want in on that action! I spent nearly a week there and during that time, I had every test and met with every specialist imaginable. At the end of the week, I was informed that without a doubt, cancer is not currently present in my body. I worked out a plan to return for scans and to remain under "surveillance" by the staff there. And, I asked about and gratefully accepted a prescription for a drug that I hope will keep cancer at bay for a while. The drug is an anti-estrogen—theoretically, the less estrogen that my body produces, the less chance there is that cancer cells will be able to feed and grow. Nothing is guaranteed, of course, but it would be silly and irresponsible for me to not explore any and all options.

My news about MDA was not greeted with the enthusiasm I had hoped for by Dr. M here in Dallas. In spite of that, he will be performing yet another surgery on me next week to remove my chemo port. I can't say that I'm excited about surgery, but I will be thrilled to have that thing out of my body! Hopefully I won't need one ever again.

With the little boys out of town for a few days, I've had time to explore a new obsession: Pinterest. PandaMom gave me a few pointers, and I am well on my way to digital organization! It makes me feel all artsy and crafty, which I am NOT in real life. Still, it's nice to imagine that one day I might be able to bake a pink heart into the center of my plain-Jane cupcakes or make a wreath out of crayons for Teacher Appreciation week.

Every year I buy Little Middle a new pair of flip flops, and every year he wears them for just a few weeks before he breaks them. Every. Single. Year. When I went to his class party on the last day of school, he was barefoot because his shoe had broken. So I gave up and I bought him a more solid, pricier pair. If they don't last him the rest of the summer, he's just gonna have to wear tennis shoes. That might have sounded heartless when I said it out loud when pulling out of the store parking lot, but Baby assured me, "You're the best mommy we could ever have." Little Middle retorted, "Yeah, but that's cause she's the ONLY mommy we can ever have."

And on that note, I'm gonna go enjoy my peace and quiet. Happy Summer!

About the Hair

Saturday, June 25, 2011

"The hair is the richest ornament of women."—Martin Luther

Fifteen months have passed since I shut my eyes tight and gripped my mom's hand as hard as I could while my hair was shaven off my head in response to chemotherapy treatments. The intense sorrow I felt during that hour at the salon was matched only by the horror I felt when I finally worked up the courage to look at myself in the mirror later that night.

They say that time heals all wounds. I disagree, but I would compromise and acknowledge that time takes the sting out of most wounds. As much as I hated it, I learned to live without my hair. Life kept going on all around me, and I made the choice to participate as much as I was able.

But my already-fragile self-esteem was shattered by my cancer-induced baldness. All these months, I've put on a brave face and a good show, but every time I looked in the mirror, I saw ugly.

Now my hair is growing. I've had it cut a few times, and recently finally got it colored because I've found that blondes really do have more fun. I begged my hairdresser to find a way to fix the crazy, kinky curls into a silky straight mane, and you know what she said? "You should embrace the curls." Humph. Some advice.

Fast forward a couple of weeks. Turns out she knows what she's talking about. After two agonizing trips and quite a few dollars to the beauty supply store, I found out that all the products and flat irons in the world can't fix this. Trying to straighten this hair only makes me look like I'm wearing a huge mushroom on my head.

So I have curls. Lots and lots of very blonde curls. I've experimented with a few different things, but the bottom line is the same every. single. day. It's still ugly. I can't comb it down or tuck it behind my ears or put a clip in it or anything. I can't even manage to make it look like I meant to style my hair this way!

Since the boys have been out of school, I have been wig-free for the most part. They have gotten used to the new look, so I know it's time for me to go public with my hair. Tomorrow will be that day. I don't mean to dramatize it, but I have great anxiety about going to church without my wig. I feel vulnerable and exposed. It's hard to explain...I think

I should feel victorious and joyful instead of scared.

I've often said I wouldn't trade my cancer journey for anything because I've learned so many valuable lessons along the way. But how I wish I could have taken this same journey with a full head of hair! But then again, what I've learned probably wouldn't have mattered nearly as much. Like knowing that life has very little to do with my hair and everything to do with my heart.

In Which I Express Myself to Cancer

Wednesday, September 28, 2011

DEAR CANCER, I HATE YOU.

I hate what you have done in my own life, and I hate that two other lives this week in my little corner of the globe were snuffed out by you.

It is your fault that these other children will grow up without mothers. It is your fault that my little boys could so easily become those children. It is your fault that those two husbands are now widowers, and I hate you so much because I have horrible dreams that my husband could be that, too. I hate you because you break families apart…good families, who love each other and love God.

I am just so mad! I am furious that you exist in the first place, and even more angry that you are so evasive. You should be cured by now, and even prevented. How are you still able to elude sophisticated medicines and scientists? Why do you insist on sneaking up on innocent people and invading their bodies? Why can't you just leave us alone?!?

Allyson Hendrickson

I despise you for making me sick, for making my hair fall out and then come back curly, for making me ration my energy and activity so I can be "normal" again, and for making me the object of pity and sympathy. I hate you for making me work so hard to figure out and trust my God—and sometimes to even question everything I have believed for most of my life.

I choose every day to beat you. I decide over and over again not to let you win. But you and I both know that you are very powerful. You have the advantage. If you decide to attack again, there's nothing I can do to change your mind.

Tomorrow morning when I wake up, I will feel—just like I do every morning—scared. But then I will choose—just like I do every morning—to not let you beat me. I will fight; I will trust.

Hear me loud and clear, Cancer: You suck. I can honestly say that I wish I had never met you. GO AWAY.

With as much sincerity as I can muster, Allyson

Trusting Jesus

Monday, October 03, 2011

I RECEIVED THIS MESSAGE FROM Little Middle's Sunday School teacher:

"...I asked the class to draw a picture of a time they had to trust Jesus. I was touched when he shared that he had to trust Jesus when you were diagnosed with cancer for the 2nd time. He's a precious boy!"

This is the picture that my Little Middle drew:

> For you are my hope; O Lord God, you are my trust from my youth and the source of my confidence. (Psalm 71:5)

Safe

Wednesday, October 12, 2011

I spent the last two days at MD Anderson testing and meeting with doctors. Today I found out that within my body, things appear to be normal. There are no "recurrent pelvic masses," no "focal suspicious bony lesions," and no "evidence of metastatic disease."

In other words, ALL CLEAR.

Tonight, I tucked my babies into their beds. I told them that Mommy is OK, and that the pictures the doctor took of my insides showed us that there is no cancer growing. To my oldest son, I said, "Even if those pictures had been different, though, it would not change the single most important thing. What is the most important thing, Goliath?" He replied, "God loves us."

And THAT is why the five of us are completely safe. Tonight, and forever.

> I will lie down and sleep in peace, for you alone, O Lord, make me dwell in safety. (Psalm 4:8)

30 Days of Thankfulness — Days 1–7

Monday, November 07, 2011

The first week of November has vanished into thin air. It's time to get caught up on my 30 days of thankfulness!

Day 1—I am thankful for the gifts of forgiveness and salvation that my Lord has given to me. I am undeserving, but He loves me so much!

Day 2—I am thankful for my Little Middle. His life and his heart are pure and simple. He loves openly and freely and doesn't expect much in return except that I love him. And I do.

Day 3—I am thankful for our house. It is cozy and roomy and…homey!

Day 4—I am thankful for my husband. We have been through so much together, but his love for me is stronger than the day we were married. I am blessed.

Day 5—I am thankful for my church. It is a place where I learn and grow, serve and give, worship and love, and receive from others. I really am glad when I go into the house of the Lord!

Day 6—I am thankful for my Bible. Hubby gave it to me for a Christmas gift the week before our first son was born. Nearly ten years later, it is worn and more than a little marked up. I don't know how I could ever replace it, though. Precious, precious book.

Day 7—I am thankful for my washing machine and dryer. I complain a lot about my laundry duties, but the reality is that every time I start a new load, I should take a minute and remember that we have SO MUCH MORE than so many people.

30 Days of Thankfulness— Days 8–9

Wednesday, November 09, 2011

DAY 8: I AM THANKFUL for the darling lady who cleans my house (no, it's not me). For a minimal wage, she comes faithfully every single Tuesday to sweep, mop, scrub, and dust all the things that I don't have time/enthusiasm for. Our agreement does not include her cleaning the little cowboys' bedrooms or their upstairs game room, but occasionally, I come home to find that she has done those rooms anyway. She is a blessing in my life.

Day 9: I am thankful for music. I often say that music is my love language. I love that when words fail me, I can find a song that expresses exactly what I feel. Back in the day, I was a diligent piano player (although my talent was debatable) and I have a history in high school marching band. I didn't grow up to be a musician, but ask my kids someday about how we blare "Sweet Caroline" in the car with the windows rolled down, or check with my friends about my "song for every occasion" quirk. Music makes memories for me.

30 Days of Thankfulness— Day 10

Thursday, November 10, 2011

Day 10: I am thankful for my country and the privilege I have to be an American citizen. I know that the freedoms I enjoy came at a price, and I am thankful for those brave men and women who sacrificed so that I can live in the greatest country in the world. One nation under God, with liberty and justice for all!

30 Days of Thankfulness— Day 11

Friday, November 11, 2011

Day 11: I am thankful for my Baby. His infectious smile and random hugs make my world go round. He loves school, he loves his friends, he loves his brothers, he loves his blue scooter and his stuffed raccoon. Being his mom has made me a better person.

30 Days of Thankfulness — Day 12

Saturday, November 12, 2011

DAY 12: I AM THANKFUL for mornings. I make it a point to get up early so I can have some quiet time before the craziness of the day begins. I love my first cup of coffee, the opportunity to spend time with God, gather my thoughts and get my bearings for the day. Every morning is a small fresh start. I am undeserving, but He is faithful.

30 Days of Thankfulness— Day 13

Sunday, November 13, 2011

DAY 13: I AM THANKFUL for my Goliath. He can be stubborn and sloppy, but his heart is tender and he loves with no limit. He is growing up SO fast! Right before my eyes, my little boy is being transformed into a young man who protects his brothers, cheers for the underdog, and loves his mom and dad. He is learning what it means to truly be a Christ-follower and how to make the right choices to walk with Jesus. He makes life an adventure—I can't wait to see what's next!

30 Days of Thankfulness — Day 14

Monday, November 14, 2011

DAY 14: I AM THANKFUL for good neighbors. We have never known our neighbors (much) until we moved into this house. I didn't really know what I was missing! I love having people close by who will help out in a childcare pinch, who will loan me pots and pans for a lasagna-making extravaganza, and who do not mind if I leave their phone number for the babysitter to use in case of an emergency. I don't have to look too far to find big blessings!

30 Days of Thankfulness— Days 15–16

Wednesday, November 16, 2011

DAY 15: I AM THANKFUL for phenergren. Seriously.

Day 16: I am thankful for all things fall. Cool temperatures, colored leaves, wind, overcast skies, pumpkin bread (and pie…and candles…). Fall is the long-awaited end of the dreadful summer season, but a breather before the rush of the holiday craze begins. To me, it's the most wonderful time of the year!

30 Days of Thankfulness — Days 17–18

Friday, November 18, 2011

DAY 17: I AM THANKFUL for my job. I love love LOVE the opportunity I have to "set the stage" for little ones to begin a lifetime of learning. We have so much fun together! ABCs and 123s are never boring with a bunch of 4-year-olds…and this particular group of littles is amazing. I love to watch them create, count, reason, play, and interact. God's goodness is evident in my classroom every week.

Day 18: I am thankful for my boys' school and their teachers. I absolutely believe that God has his hand over my children each year when they start school, and maybe never more so than now. My sons are blessed with amazing, dedicated professionals who want them to succeed academically, but also care for their spirits. Goliath, Little Middle, and Baby love school! God did that, and I am grateful.

30 Days of Thankfulness— Days 19–24

Thursday, November 24, 2011

DAY 19: I AM THANKFUL for my grandparents. I have been blessed with amazing relationships with them that a lot of people never get to have. I count the four of them among my very favorite people, and many of my happiest memories involve them. I like to imagine that my Grandad is spending his time in eternity building beautiful things to put in the family mansions so he can show off to the rest of us when we get there. I still miss him every day. Gran, Buck, Grandmama~I love you so much!

Day 20: I am thankful for my "Tuesday Sisters" Bible study group. We have met, in some form, for more than 10 years. This is a core group of friends and sisters in Christ who I am privileged to do life with. They have prayed for me, laid hands on me, pushed me to be better, let me complain and/or cry when I needed to. We eat, we shop, we study, and we laugh. We laugh a LOT. They are faithful friends, and I wouldn't be the woman I am without them.

Day 21: I am thankful for Caroline. Caroline has been my friend for as long as I can remember. She knows things about me that no one else knows. She was my first sleepover buddy, it was her fault that I got my name written on the board in 3rd grade, and she was the one who shared my excitement when that special boy finally kissed me as a teenager (turns out he wasn't really that special after all). She was my maid of honor and I was hers. We have shared joys and heartaches. A friendship like ours is something that not everyone gets to have. She is my lifelong bucket-filler…how fortunate am I?

Day 22: I am thankful for my brother. He was kind of a pest when we were kids, but he turned out to be a pretty cool guy. His quick wit and unique perspective on life make me think and often make me laugh. He loves music, people, and animals. Most of all, he loves God and seeks to walk with Him hand in hand.

Day 23: I am thankful for my sister. Despite our age difference, we have always had a close relationship, but the older we get, the better friends we become. I count her among my closest friends. She is funny, she is stylish, she is sweet, and sometimes she is righteously indignant. She "gets" me, and I adore her.

Day 24: I am thankful for my parents. If you have never met my mom and dad, you are missing out! Today is their 38th wedding anniversary. They love each other, and together they taught us what love is. I am so grateful for their example of commitment and loyalty to each other and to family. They way they live has helped shape me as a wife and a mother, and set the standard for what I want for my children.

30 Days of Thankfulness— Day 25

Friday, November 25, 2011

DAY 25: I AM THANKFUL for AbbyDog. I will never ever forget when Abby came into my life. She was a tiny puppy whose ears were bigger than the rest of her body. We lived in a loft apartment (we were carefree newlyweds) and Abby couldn't climb the stairs because she would trip on her ears! She has been through five moves and three babies with us and never complained. When I was sick, she would lay in bed with me. On my darkest, most scary days, when I wanted to cover my head and never come out, my princess puppy was there loving me. She follows me everywhere I go, and she always is glad to see me when I come home. I love my dog!

30 Days of Thankfulness — Day 26

Saturday, November 26, 2011

DAY 26: I AM THANKFUL for the joy I feel as the holiday season begins. Last year, I asked God desperately for a glimmer of hope, a restoration of joy. My body was weary and my spirit depleted. What a difference a year makes! I felt it as I decorated my in-laws' Christmas tree with Baby last night, and I feel it as I am looking forward to decorating my own home this weekend. I have always loved this time of year; I hated it so much last year that happiness felt just beyond my grasp. I am blessed beyond measure, and thankful.

30 Days of Thankfulness — Days 27–29

Tuesday, November 29, 2011

Day 27: I am thankful for good food. I like to spend time in my kitchen, perusing my collection of cookbooks and planning meals for my family. I am grateful that I enjoy cooking and that every resource I need is readily available to me. So many people in so many places could only dream about the food that I consume every single day.

Day 28: I am thankful simply that the five people that live in this house are a family. We are not perfect by any means, but we love each other and we are intact. None of us are guaranteed tomorrow. So we work to take care of each other. We fight for what really matters. We say "I love you." My whole world is wrapped up under this roof.

Day 29: I am thankful for my bed. It is the most comfy, cozy place in the world! Once the boys are in bed, I retreat to our bedroom for some "me" time. Some nights I read, some nights I watch TV. I have a safe, warm place to relax and sleep every night. People in my own community don't have what I have.

30 Days of Thankfulness— Day 30

Wednesday, November 30, 2011

DAY 30: I AM THANKFUL that I have so much to be thankful for. It may sound a little silly, but this month I have been intentional about counting my blessings, and I have not once found it difficult to be grateful. What I have, who I'm with, where I live… these are the blessings that God has poured out on me. My life is a testament to His goodness. I don't deserve anything at all, but He is the giver of all good things.

Miracle to Miracle

Saturday, December 31, 2011

I ACCOMPLISHED—AND LEARNED—A LOT IN 2011. In the last 12 months, I:

- fulfilled a life dream and met Mary Poppins.
- sought and found help at M.D. Anderson.
- finished a year's worth of chemotherapy and Avastin treatments.
- moved into my perfect house. How I love it here!
- mourned the loss of two precious unborn babies.
- went to about a thousand little boy birthday parties.
- sweltered through the hottest summer EVER.
- continued to study, learn, and grow with my Tuesday Sisters.
- grew my hair back!
- made some new friends in our neighborhood and through the boys' school.
- realized that mothering is not for the faint of heart when Goliath went to camp for a week and later competed in a martial arts tournament.

- went hunting with my man. After 13 years of marriage, it's about time.
- tolerated and even learned to love Gus the Terrible.
- found my inner crafter and spent a lot of time and money at Hobby Lobby.
- discovered Pinterest.
- buried a deceased bunny rabbit and welcomed our guinea pigs' love child into our menagerie.
- went to Disney World, the circus, and a snake farm.

> To be alive, to be able to see, to walk…it's all a miracle. I have adopted the technique of living life from miracle to miracle.
>
> —Arthur Rubinstein

New Year's Eve is not really a big deal to us. We used to try to stay up late to watch the ball drop; now we're too old and have too many kids to care. When I wake up in the morning, 2012 will have begun. I won't eat black-eyed peas, I won't hum "Auld Lang Syne," and I won't make resolutions. Instead, I will begin tomorrow like I begin every morning: choosing to LIVE my life. Not too many people get the opportunity that I have had to examine life and re-discover what is truly important. Every single day that I wake up is a miracle. Every experience, every encounter, every minute…miracles. Instead of making temporary resolutions, I want to make one permanent promise to myself: I will recognize my life's miracles and soak them up. I will make the most of what I've been given to be the best me that I can be.

Here's to a 2012 full of grace and love…Happy New Year!

Bullet Briefing

Saturday, January 28, 2012

- Blogging has taken a backseat on my priority list lately. These bullet points are all I can muster, I'm afraid.
- A 36-hour trip to Houston last week resulted in clean scans. The anxiety leading up to that trip can not be accurately described except to tell you that I was popping Xanax like candy. The relief I felt after the trip is equally indescribable.
- I flew Southwest for my trip. Not only was I "randomly selected" for extra security measures (read: You might be a terrorist, so we are going to humiliate you in front of hundreds of strangers.), but one of my shoes fell out of the bin when it went through the x-ray machine. While standing on one foot so as not to contaminate my bare foot, I summoned an officer for help. She had to stop the conveyor belt, hold up the line, and climb up on to the belt to retrieve my missing shoe.
- God gave me this verse on the day I went to M.D. Anderson: "You, O Lord, are a shield around me. You are my glory, and the lifter of my head." Psalm 3:3

- While I was lying on the table during my test, trying not to freak out, I was reciting that verse over and over to myself. Halfway through the test, the little tech man entered the room and said to me, "You're doing great. Now for the next part I need to put this shield over you." I started to cry. He looked puzzled, and I suppose he thought I didn't understand. He said, "It's okay, ma'am. The shield is for protection." I know, sir. I know.
- I had several hours to kill between tests, so my mom and I left the hospital and went over to Hermann Park to ride the train. It's been 20+ years since I did that! I loved it just as much as a grown woman as I did when I was a little girl.
- My dad comes to M.D. Anderson when I meet with my doctor to get test results. In the absence of my Hubby, who is home taking care of our cowboys, I feel very safe. It takes a good man to sit in the gynecological oncology waiting room.
- Our Sunday School class came over to our house last weekend and we played Headbanz. Just because it says "5 and up" on the box doesn't mean adults can't play.
- Some people look more foolish than others wearing Headbanz cards on their heads.
- I am learning how to play Mexican train. Hubby has never played before in his life, and when we played with friends, he won. I don't know how he pulled that off.
- Baby read "Goodnight, Moon" to me at bedtime the other night. It made me cry.
- Baby read "Old Hat, New Hat" to me last night. He wants to practice so he can take it to school and read it in front of his class.
- The boys now have assigned seats in my car. They drive me crazy sometimes.

- I thought it would be nice of me to volunteer to take a turn hosting Little Middle's cub scout den meeting. Two things I have to say about that: the den leaders are saints, and we will probably never do it again.
- As soon as the last scout was out the door, I put on my slippers and went next door for a girls' night in. My darling neighbor was generous with her wine and her company, and I immediately felt better. Especially when I saw that her refrigerator AND her stove were in her living room due to kitchen remodeling. It's the only time that my house will ever be tidier than hers.
- Baby is sitting next to me right now singing "Dynamite."
- Little Middle raced a car in his first pinewood derby. It didn't go that well. :(
- I bought my unborn niece her first pair of shoes today and a bib that says "I Love My Auntie." Indeed she will.
- My mom, my sister, my SIL, and I are planning a girls' trip for the first part of Spring Break. Can. Not. Wait.
- I miss my grandparents.
- My co-teacher and I hosted a "Pre-K Preview" day last week in our classroom for parents who are considering sending their children to us next year. All things considered, I think it went well.
- Cotton candy was invented in 1904 and used to be called fairy floss. Thank you, Food Network.
- Hubby plays Words With Friends with my aunt, and he is in awe of her WWF skillz.
- My dad and my uncle are going to the Master's. I am so happy for my daddy, because he will get to check something off of his bucket list.
- I think I really want to see "Extremely Loud and Incredibly Close." Then again, I am a little scared to see it.
- The boys and I watch "Call of the Wildman" every week together. If you haven't seen it, you should catch it on

Animal Planet. There is nothing more backwoods than the Turtle Man.
- I am learning that I can't protect the people I love from other people who might hurt them, and that hurts me.
- Some mornings I play Phil Joel's "Good Morning" to wake the boys up for school. One morning, Little Middle rolled over and growled at me, "I would rather put SCISSORS in my EARS than listen to you sing this song to me!!!!" Every time I think of him saying that, I giggle.
- Last weekend Goliath cleaned out my car, including vacuuming. Five days later, I spilled a whole cup of coffee in there and had to get the upholstery professionally cleaned.
- I have had fun lately downloading new fonts to use with my Word documents. So nerdy.
- I think about what it would be like if I die. Not for me, but for my family. I go back and forth on whether I would want Hubby to remarry. I certainly want him—all of them—to be happy, but I don't like the thought that I could be replaced.
- I am an emotional eater.
- My bed is the most comfy place in the whole world.
- I got tall black boots for Christmas, and I love them!
- Someone told me the other day that I am well-dressed. I don't know about that, but I appreciated the compliment.
- Hubby changed his ringer on his phone. Now when I call him, his phone plays "Pretty Woman." Aw.
- Sometimes I listen to the song "How He Loves Us" by the David Crowder Band, and I am overwhelmed. If His grace is an ocean, we're all sinking.

At the Heart of the Matter

Monday, February 20, 2012

AT BEDTIME...

Baby: Mommy, I am worried about you.
Me: What are you worried about?
Baby: I am worried that you don't feel good.
Me: Baby, Mommy is fine right now. Do you mean you are worried that I will get sick again?
Baby: Yes. I feel sad about that, Mom.

This is just one of the things that burdens my heart right now. But it is by far the heaviest: the fear that follows us—even the smallest of us—everywhere we go.

> How long must I wrestle with my thoughts and day after day have sorrow in my heart? How long will the enemy triumph over me? Look on me and answer, Lord my God. (Psalm 13:2–3)

Dwelling in the Desert, Part 1

Friday, April 13, 2012

There is a "travel challenge" making its way around Facebook. It lists the top 100 places you should visit, and then I suppose you see how much traveling you still ought to do before you die and you feel bad about it. I haven't done that challenge, but I carry a mental list of places I want to go: Italy and Jerusalem with my husband, Washington D.C. with my kids, London and New York with my mom and sister, Las Vegas with my friends. One place definitely not on my list is the desert. It's SO hot. Weird creatures live there. It's wide open and it's scary. I don't wanna go. But somehow, I landed smack dab in the middle of a desert anyway. I had no intention of going there. It wasn't on my calendar or on my "to-do" list. I've been there for a while now. And I'm here to tell you that it is every bit as uncomfortable and unpleasant as I thought it might be. My desert, of course, is a different sort than what comes to mind when you think "Sahara." My desert is emotional, a little bit physical, and very, very spiritual. I woke up one Friday morning in February and

    I couldn't get out of bed. I wasn't sick, at least not physically. I cried for no reason. I could not bring myself to do the simple everyday things that make my world go round. I didn't cook. I didn't hang out with my boys. I didn't hang up clothes or run errands or drive the kids to activities or write lesson plans or call friends or wash my hair or anything. For three days I stayed in bed. It was the only place I felt safe. My sweet Hubby took over my responsibilities and allowed me that time to be sad and scared. On Monday, I knew that I had to get back to life whether I felt like it or not. I also knew that my heart was sick and that I needed help. I found help with a Christian counselor who I've been seeing for several months. At our first meeting, she just let me talk. Well, to be honest, she asked me a bunch of questions that I answered honestly but quickly. See, I have a "safe zone" when it comes to talking about myself and especially when asking for help. My husband, my parents, and a few close friends are in the zone. Pouring out my deepest thoughts to a total stranger took my anxiety level through the roof. Telling her about everything was unbelievably hard. "Everything" includes, but is certainly not limited to The Sickness and how it has turned my life 100% upside down. (There are other issues, of course, that are ongoing and un-blog-able.) Cancer came out of nowhere and knocked me down to the ground. Then, just when I was getting my second wind and was trying to move on, it took me down again. It moved on, but I believe that it is just temporary. Now I know that it is after me and that I can be blindsided at any time. It takes an enormous amount of effort to pretend that I'm fine, to act normal, to keep my worry and sorrow to myself, and most of all, to protect my family. Basically, I am killing myself trying to control something that I have absolutely no control over whatsoever. And, in the back of my mind and in the deepest part of my heart, there is a little nagging voice saying, "Where is God?" For the first time in my entire life, I couldn't find Him. "Why, O Lord, do you stand far off? Why do you hide yourself in times of trouble?" (Ps. 10:1)

Heavy

Wednesday, July 18, 2012

THE THREE LITTLE COWBOYS AND I are at kids' camp with our church this week. The people, the worship, and the teaching are fantastic. The food is questionable; the weather is hot. Both of those were to be expected.

On this day, my heart is heavy. Precious leaders in our church who I have been privileged to count among my friends moved halfway across the country to serve another church just weeks ago. This morning their fourth child, a daughter, was born. Baby Blake has a severe heart malfunction and she remains in critical condition, her hours-old life hanging in the balance.

My cousin is the mother to a darling five-year-old girl who suffers from a rare muscular disease. Her enzyme levels skyrocketed today, and she has been admitted to the hospital. Each "episode" that Ellia has is life-threatening.

I had a regularly-scheduled CT scan a couple of weeks ago. I received an "all clear," only to have the doctor and radiologist re-read the film and find a small mass. I will have a biopsy done on Monday to determine what it is and what to do about it.

There is another situation happening within my home that is too large and too hard to put out there just yet. I am in a place that is isolating and terribly frightening. My three boys are why I get out of bed each morning and give it my best, in spite of my fear. rippling fear.

And then, in a worship service in the middle of nowhere surrounded by hundreds of children, God gave me a song. He promises to do that, you know: "He put a new song in my mouth, a hymn of praise to our God." Psalm 40:3

I am begging him for favor and mercy for myself, and for those who are close to my heart. He is able, and He is good.

Update

Monday, July 23, 2012

Two days before we went to camp, my Plan B oncologist (the one I see when/if I can't get to MDA in Houston) discovered a suspicious spot during a routine follow-up physical exam. He actually referred to it as a "nodule," which I think in medical speak covers a multitude of possibilities. Today I had a CT-guided biopsy of that nodule so we can find out what it is and what to do about it. The procedure went well, except for the part when the radiologist told me that there were several spots of concern. I might have panicked except for two things: 1. I knew that God is in control of everything, however many nodules there may be, and 2. The sedation meds kicked in just when the doctor finished his last sentence.

The radiology report will be completed within 24 hours, but the pathology results will take a couple of days. I plan to meet with my doctor on Thursday morning to get those results. Friends and strangers alike are praying faithfully for favorable results, and I am grateful. "When I am afraid, I will put my trust in You" (Psalm 56:3).

Results

Wednesday, July 25, 2012

Twenty-four hours ago I was at the swimming pool with my kids, just enjoying them. Right now I am sitting in my living room trying to wrap my head around the news I got today: I have cancer. It's back. In three places.

I will meet with my dr. here in Dallas tomorrow morning; test results and reports are being sent to my team at M.D. Anderson. We will decide what to do, although I am told that surgery may not be an option and chemotherapy almost certainly is.

What in the world will I say to my sons? Christ, have mercy.

Courage from Cowboys

Friday, July 27, 2012

Thursday, July 26 will go down in history as one of the most wretched days of my entire life. That's saying something, because I've had more than my fair share of bad days!

First was a visit to Dr. F, my Plan B oncologist. He confirmed the presence of serous papillary carcinoma (read: $&#;%! cancer) in three different spots in my pelvic region. He went on to say that there is some uncertainty among the medical team if those three spots are the only spots. The harsh truth is that by the time a patient has a third recurrence, their body tends to be filled with cancer. Three different radiologists have looked at my CT film, and they do not entirely agree on what is going on in there.

To that end, I will have a PET scan next week. Hopefully the radioactive material will light up those awful cells and reveal their hiding places.

Dr. F suggested that surgery probably will not be an option. The data for third-time cancer surgeries is limited at best, and any data that is available is probably for women twice my age. Given the location of the known masses, the surgery would be risky for interference with a few organs and their functions.

Three Little Cowboys

Chemotherapy is a must, and the sooner I get started, the better. I am looking at a Taxol/carboplatin combination, every 3 weeks for six rounds. The timing here is very important. Each cancerous mass has the ability to double in size in as few as 30 days. 18 weeks of chemo leads us straight into the holidays, at which time there will be another round of scans to determine what, if anything, needs to happen differently.

That's the medical, practical side of this thing. It's dry and it's terrifying…but compared to the terror I felt as I sat across from my little cowboys, it is nothing. First, I gave them the good news: Mom loves you very much and there's nothing you can do about it. Then, the bad news: Mom has new cancer growing in her body.

Immediate panic ensued, especially for Goliath. I had just given life to his worst fear.

The only thing I care to remember about that conversation yesterday is how they all reacted with fierce emotion. They are each so wonderfully unique, so Goliath's breathlessness=Little Middle's hung head=Baby's tears. As much as I detest the bad news that turned life upside down for my sons in that instant, I love that their reaction demonstrates how they love me. If nothing else goes right from here on out, I will remember that they are scared and emotional because I am important to them. It's a terrible, but somewhat comforting, thought.

I answered their questions as best I could, and reminded them what is really important:

Cancer doesn't change God. God loves us just as much today as He did yesterday. God isn't surprised, even though we sure are. God knows that we're angry, and He understands. We can make a choice to trust Him or to stay angry.

This morning, on the way to an appointment, Goliath and I cut through the high school parking lot. We rolled down the car windows and started yelling: "I HATE CANCER!"

"CANCER STINKS!" Construction workers turned their heads, but we didn't care. We felt better.

Somehow, I will make it okay for my boys to yell. I will encourage them to express their distaste for this horrid disease that has reared its ugly head once again. I will do everything possible to make sure they know that they are THE reasons I will fight, and fight I will. I will tell them and show them that I love them. I WILL NOT DIE. God gave me one life—one chance—to be their mom. The cowboys give me courage.

I am waiting to be able to talk with Dr. B, my Plan A/M.D. Anderson doc. She and Dr. F will put their heads together to make final decisions about treatment. Unless she offers a miracle experimental drug that can only come from MDA, I plan to remain close to home for treatment. I will update early next week as plans are finalized.

I wish I could understand, but I don't. I wish I had a glimpse of the big picture, but it eludes me. What I am sure of is this: He is close. As long as I am able, I will run to Him.

Coming Up...

Tuesday, July 31, 2012

Dr. F called last night. The PET scan showed that the cancer is contained in my abdomen/pelvis. A big concern had been that cancerous cells had spread to the liver and/or lungs, but it's just not there! Based on those results, Dr. F, along with Dr. B of M.D. Anderson fame, has decided to operate. I will go into surgery on Monday morning to have all three masses removed. The surgery will include a colon resection, similar to what I experienced in 2010.

After the surgery, I can expect to spend a week—maybe a little more—in the hospital (it was a 9-day stay last time—entirely too long, in my opinion). During my recovery, my medical team will send the tumors off for chemo sensitivity testing. This process involves treating pieces of the tumor with chemotherapy drugs and watching the effect: do they shrink? do they remain the same? This is how Dr. F will know whether or not to treat me with chemo, and which drugs may be most effective. I am not holding out much hope that this means no chemo at all for me, but I am encouraged that if I have to do it, I will be taking the right meds for my specific cancer growth.

Allyson Hendrickson

The little cowboys have been informed of the surgery. Here's a little bit of that conversation:

Goliath: How do they get the cancer out, Mom? LittleMiddle: The doctor cuts Mom's stomach and takes it out. Me: That's right, buddy. When he does that… Goliath: Yeah, but how does he DO it? Does he have really sharp scissors? LittleMiddle: No, he uses a knife. I think it's like the one that Dad used to kill that wild hog at the lease.

They don't like the idea that I will be away from them, and neither do I! I am asking God to put a kind, super-compassionate nurse in place that might let them sneak in to visit.

In the meantime, we are soaking up every available minute we have together. They don't know that I am scared, they don't know that I wrestle with God. What they do know is that their mom loves them. And somehow, for this hot summer afternoon, that seems to be enough.

You Alone

Sunday, August 05, 2012

IT IS LATE AND MY house is quiet. The cowboys are safely (and dare I say happily?) sleeping over with friends. Abby Dog is resting by my feet. On any other night, I would feel content.

Tonight, though, I am a tornado of emotions and anxiety and fear. When I wake up in the morning, I will shower and head to the hospital. I will walk the now-familiar halls down to the surgical wing. I will kiss my husband, hug my parents, wave to our friends, and bravely—I hope—go back to the operating room.

This summer, particularly these last few weeks, has been so hard. It seems that even when I try to stand very still, the world continues to crumble around me. My best efforts to hold it all together have failed miserably. I have witnessed so much suffering, not the least of which is my own. The pain and loss that I feel is nearly unbearable. Nearly. And just when I am teetering on the edge, literally fearing for my life, my Jesus calls out to me. He reminds me of his goodness. He reminds me that I don't have to be scared. He reminds me that he goes with me and that he loves me.

You alone, Lord, are enough. Thank you for holding me close tonight. May my weakness be perfected in your strength.

Hospital, Day 5

Saturday, August 11, 2012

Days in the hospital are L-O-N-G. The day started out behind the curve when morning light revealed that I looked like I felt: like I'd been run over by a big truck. See, there's this funny thing about getting your whole body cut apart and re-pieced back together—the body has to teach itself how to work again. The way that God created our bodies is an amazing thing. According to Dr. F, my body will bounce back from 3 invasive tumors and a resectioned (again) colon to become just as functional as it was before. It simply takes time.

So while I'm waiting, I want you to know that I appreciate you. Thank you for taking time to check up on me. Thank you for the care that you've shown to me and my family, and for faithfully praying. I need a clear head to try to truly communicate my heart to you…that will come later, when all of the parts are in working order again! For now, know that the encouragement you've shown me force me to look ahead and your prayers spur my own faith. Thank you.

Hospital, Day 6

Sunday, August 12, 2012

Today I...

- shaved my legs (the parts I could reach, anyway).
- got to wear pretty pink pjs in place of the icky hospital gown.
- continued to wonder how Ryan Seacrest belongs both on American Idol and the Olympics.
- ate a saltine, some ice cream, and a few bites of baked potato.
- drank apple juice.
- had a nice fireside chat with Dr. F. I still can't believe that a doctor actually cares so much about his patients that he will spend hours just talking about cancer and also revealing that he only carries a beer around at parties because his wife makes him.
- listened to a brand new baby crying. The post-natal floor is full, so they are moving some patients up here.
- got to visit with a few friends, both new and old.

- got to hug my cowboys and let them push the buttons on the bed to move up and down. Smile.
- was disconnected from a couple of machines and switched from fluid to oral meds. Progress!
- missed being in church, but told God "thank you" for giving me such a great church to miss.
- talked through some things with Mom and Dad. Told God "thank you" for these two amazing people whose unconditional love keeps me going.
- received pictures of Tex the Nephew Dog and Reese the Niece that made me smile.
- marvelled that at this time last week, I was physically whole. Thought about how God takes broken things and put them back together, and knew that in another week I will be marvelling again.
- watched the Olympics closing ceremony with my dad. Couldn't figure out the weird octopus with the d.j. in the middle spinning tunes.

No Place Like Home

Thursday, August 16, 2012

I GOT TO COME HOME unexpectedly early on Monday night. My sweet dad battled crazy Dallas traffic for over an hour, but it was well worth it when he delivered me to this:

Yep, those are my guys being glad to see me. And me, sporting crazy hospital hair, even more glad to see them.

Within the first 12 hours of being home, I broke one of the many rules that Dr. F had laid out for me: avoid the stairs. I seem to think that I am younger and in better shape than what I am, thereby being exempt from silly rules. All I can say now is that the boys better keep their rooms clean, because I will not be going upstairs to check on them for some time. Speaking of keeping our rooms clean…did you know that if you are living under this roof and you are in the 10-and-under age bracket, you can earn real $$$ by keeping your room clean? We call it a random room check (or RRC, for short, per Goliath). The RRC is the brainchild of Nana, who has moved in temporarily to do my jobs so I can rest and recover. RRC is a big hit with my cowboys!

My mother…I want so much to tell you what it means to me that she is here in my home. I want to tell you how I am amazed at how she keeps up with all the little boy laundry—something I am never able to do myself!—, keeps the kitchen spotless, and makes it all look easy. I want to communicate how her unconditional love and sacrifice makes me feel like I am the most important person in the world and how her presence here comforts me. I want to make you understand that The Sickness is just a part of the curve ball life has thrown at me this summer, and that she helps me navigate my way and feel hopeful that it will be okay. I wish I could explain how my sons have security and even a sense of normalcy because their Nana is caring for them. Words are simply insufficient. I have been overwhelmed lately with what I have in my life that is abnormal and faulty. But when it comes to my mom, I can't help but be overwhelmingly thankful, because I know that I have something in her that many people never get to have, and she blesses me beyond measure.

It is worth noting here also that my hospital stay ended just in the nick of time. This was my second stay on the 9th floor at MCD, and I think that my familiarity entitles me to make customer suggestions. My first suggestion will be that there be some sort of discount off the overall hospital bill for patients who are able to do awesome medical tricks, i.e. remove an epidural line that is inserted and taped to your back, or remove a 4-foot NG tube that was running from your nose down to your stomach. Extra dollars off should be rewarded for doing it in the shower without being aware of it. I will be looking for those discounts on my next statement.

Abby Dog's birthday quietly came and went while I was in the hospital. She is now 14 and 98 years old (human and dog years, respectively). I felt bad that she didn't get her usual family party, but maybe we can make up for it once I'm back on my feet. Honestly, she is so geriatric that I doubt she missed it much. The old girl remains my most faithful friend with the biggest ears. Love her.

Three Little Cowboys

Goliath and Baby are delighted that the first day of school is fast-approaching—come on, Monday, August 27th!!—while Little Middle is mourning the summer days that are slipping away. Thankfully, I listened to a smart friend last spring who has 3 boys of her own and offered me this advice: "Buy the wrap packs, Allyson. The boys don't care about the shopping. Buy the wrap packs!" School supplies will be there waiting on the first day.

Backpacks and lunch boxes were purchased before I went to the hospital. Nana is filling in the blanks and is helping the boys get their back-to-school style ready. My Goliath has a definite idea about what a 5th grade boy's clothes should be; in one word: cool. Don't tell my mom, but I'm a little glad she is doing this shopping trip with him. My mommy-heart might not be able to handle the coolness of my little boy.

Although he is younger, Baby is also making choices regarding his own style. He is replacing his old athletic shoes with these:

Sniff. So cute. And grown-up.

My Little Middle, however, hates shopping. He would rather eat a vegetable casserole for breakfast than have to be dragged on a shopping trip, even if it is for his own clothes and shoes. In a nice arrangement that can only be made if your grandmother lives to make you happy, he has simply described to Nana what he wants to wear on the first day of school. She is going to shop for him and bring it home. He's happy because he doesn't have to go to a real store, and she's happy because she doesn't have to hunt for him in all the clothes racks. Problem solved.

And while the family does their thing, I am carefully nursing my long row of abdominal staples and working to keep food where it belongs. It's a glamorous life, I tell you. It will be another week or so before I know any results from chemo sensitivity testing. Until then, I plan to take it easy and soak up the goodness that surrounds me. There really is no place like home.

The Sickness: Chapter 3

Wednesday, August 29, 2012

Yesterday I met the Top 6 Most Annoying People on the Planet. They were all in the oncology waiting room at MCD. I had plenty of time to figure out how annoying they were, because I waited over 2 hours to get to see the doctor. I seriously doubt that 1) the upcoming presidential election can fix health care, and 2) that the disabled woman really had a hemi engine in her wheelchair like her bumper sticker claimed. Dr. F said that my incision is healing nicely. Although I still don't feel great, I am learning more every day about my new-and-not-so-improved insides. It is a delicate balance of food and meds that will be tolerated. Anything outside those imaginary boundaries is quickly rejected by my body and I pay the price for days. Dr. F assures me that I will feel better, but it will take time. Time as in months, not as in days. I was also released to drive a car and climb stairs as I feel that I am able. That means more freedom, which I have sorely missed! Last night, I went upstairs and tucked my cowboys into bed for the first time in three weeks. Smile. Then we moved on to the "what comes next" phase of the visit. One of the two chemosensitivity tests have come back. Dr. F gave me the stack of papers marked "FINAL REPORT" in big, bold letters. At first, I didn't understand what I was looking at.

But as he began to talk, I began to absorb information. On one side of the cover page of the report, there is a column that lists 13 different drugs, or families of related drugs, that are labeled "Agents Associated With Potential Lack of Benefit." It means just what it says—each medicine listed there is ineffective in my body to fight cancer. The list includes Taxol and Cisplatin, the two chemo drugs that rocked my world less than 2 years ago. You can not imagine the sick feeling in the pit of my stomach. There is another list on the other side of the page labeled "Agents Associated With Potential Benefit." There is 1 drug listed there. ONE. There is ONE chemotherapy drug that might help me. I felt like I'd been punched in the gut. I had gone in to this office visit believing that I had choices. I was prepared to accept chemo, but I was also prepared to reject it if this test showed that the compatible chemo drugs were too harsh. I believed that I was entitled to choose for myself. It never entered my mind that I wouldn't have options. And I didn't even need to ask Dr. F what would happen if I don't do the chemo. I already know. I went through hell, and it didn't matter. I can barely wrap my mind around it. I see now that I have no choices. I have to do the chemotherapy. It's one drug…one chance…my only chance. This has to work, or… STOP. The drug is Doxil. It is a cytotoxic drug that is used to treat aggressive forms of ovarian cancer and a specific type of sarcoma that is related to the AIDS virus. That mental image is sobering. Doxil is an irritant. Side effects and their severity depend on how much of the drug is received. Possible side effects include low blood counts (increased risk for infection), skin rash, hand-foot syndrome, peeling and/or sores on the skin, nausea, vomiting, hair thinning and/or loss, poor appetite, stomach/digestive issues. Those are the main ones. There is also a risk of interference with the pumping action of the heart. My heart will be closely monitored for signs of disease or decreased efficiency at pumping blood. If everything goes right, I will have my first Doxil infusion next Thursday. I will do one infusion every four weeks for six cycles, with the last one in February. We will do a CT scan in November and again in February to check progress. I have found that past chemotherapy has left my veins in terrible shape, so I will be required to have another port put in. We are still unsure when that surgery will be.

> My heart is in anguish within me; the terrors of death have fallen on me. Fear and trembling have beset me; horror has overwhelmed me. I said, "Oh, that I had the wings of a dove! I would fly away and be at rest. I would flee far away and stay in the desert; I would hurry to my place of shelter, far from the tempest and the storm." (Psalm 55:4–8)

Tidbits

Tuesday, September 04, 2012

- I had an echocardiogram last week to set a baseline for chemo treatments. The tech told me that my aorta is "pretty."
- I went to a chemo teaching session. Doxil is a strong drug, but not as toxic as the Taxol/Cisplatin regimen that I did 2 years ago. I am on high alert for hand-foot syndrome, symptoms of anemia, fever, and mouth sores. It is anticipated that my hair will thin, but will not all fall out as before.
- Chemo starts on Thursday.
- Before the chemo infusion begins, I will have surgery to put a port in place. Yes, on the same day. I have to check in with day surgery at 5:45 a.m.
- Today is the first day of preschool. I just can't believe I'm not there with my little friends! In spite of my best efforts, I feel very sad that I am missing out. adorable.
- Hubby took all of the cowboys out to the lease for the opening weekend of dove season. In their absence, I got

to have a girls' weekend with my sister and Reese the Niece! We ate warm tortillas from Rosa's, watched girl movies, stayed in our pajamas, and played with the baby. Goodness, I love that little girl!

- With chemo starting, I have a conundrum. I have been putting off getting my hair done because I was anticipating losing it again. Now that I know with a fair amount of certainty that at least some of it will stay, I need to do something about those roots. Unfortunately, my nurse advised me to avoid hair coloring. The reaction of the chemicals in the dye with the poisonous chemicals in the drug may exacerbate the hair thinning. On the other hand, it's already looking pretty neglected. I'm hoping that there may be something natural to use in the interim to give me the color that I want without burning up whatever hair I get to keep.
- Last night while he was in the shower, Little Middle said to Hubby, "Can I shave? It's on my bucket list!"
- Baby has already had more homework than both of his brothers combined. For one project, he had to make a paper doll of himself. For another, he had to cut pictures out of magazines and decorate his daily journal cover with them so he can have inspiration for writing. Um, how much inspiration does a six-year-old need?
- Goliath has an appointment with the eye doctor this afternoon. He has been complaining about blurred vision, especially now that school has started back up. I will not be surprised at all if he needs glasses. He is worried, but I think he would be.
- Adorable is not cool in the 5th grade. 5th graders also do not "play," they "hang out." Just sayin'.

Doxil 1/6

Thursday, September 06, 2012

Today was my first day of Doxil chemotherapy. All things considered, it went fairly well. Mom and I stayed in a hotel close to the hospital last night because of the ungodly hour I had to be there this morning. In spite of the massive construction project on 635, we got there on time. It's funny how the surgery protocol is old hat to me. The first time I had surgery at MCD, we got lost in the hospital and I remember well feeling like I would throw up from anxiety. This morning, I knew exactly where to go, what to expect, and even knew a few surgery nurses by name. My favorite nurse, Cynthia, was my pre-admit nurse when I had my major procedure 2 years ago. She said, "It's back? Well, CRAP." That just about says it all. I opted to do the surgery with minimal anesthesia. I did not want to feel very groggy or have to spend time in the recovery room. The anesthesiologist gave me a "margarita" of drugs and they injected numbing meds around the site. It's a very odd feeling to be aware of someone cutting you open. I am in more pain now than I was during the surgery, although I remember saying "ouch" a few times. I was wheeled straight from surgery to chemo. My chemotherapy is administered in a large room that can fit 10 patients at a time. There are partition walls between each recliner chair, giving the false sense of privacy. At least I don't have to look at everyone, or worse, endure them looking at me. Pre-meds were minimal, only fluids and an anti-nausea drug. The Doxil itself is red. Kool-Aid red, homemade Valentines red. The shade of red that made me think of happy celebrations instead of a wretched bag of life-saving poison. I was wishing so much that I had a bouquet of balloons and a cake with delicious butter cream frosting instead of bruised skin and an unshakable headache! Mom and I tried to watch a movie together on the TV screen that was provided, but a very unhappy patient across the room dragged her IV pole over and asked us to keep it down. Humph. The woman at the station next to me asked the nurse if her friend could grab a snack from the stash they keep for patients. Although the nurse made it clear that the food was for chemo patients only, the friend went ahead and gave the nurse her order: peanut butter crackers and cranberry juice. If they didn't have cranberry, she would settle for grape juice, but was obviously displeased. They then carried on an in-depth theological discussion for the remainder of the afternoon that was just loud enough for the rest of us to hear. The good news is that there is a fish tank in the room. Worst case scenario, I can watch the fish. Even with all of that, we still made it home before the cowboys got off the school bus. I feel…well, I don't feel crummy. I feel very tired and sore and a little bit sad. But my cowboys—they came in like nothing was wrong. They talked to their Nana and hugged their mom and I knew. I KNEW that I am doing the right thing, even though it is hard. I would have rather been a hundred other places today than at that hospital, but at the end of the day, I am their mom. I laughed at Goliath's story that he told about his friends, I helped Little Middle study for his spelling test tomorrow (who knew that "unusual" would give him so much trouble?!?), and I listened to Baby read Green Eggs and Ham to me. It's his favorite. Those three little boys are all my favorites.

As this day comes to an end, I realize that I have experienced God's mercy, grace, and kindness in a thousand different ways. Hundreds—literally hundreds—of people prayed for me and my family today. Knowing that simply blows my mind. I came in contact with helpful and compassionate doctors, nurses, and staff who made a hard day easier for me. My sons are healthy and happy. "He told me, 'My grace is enough; it's all you need. My strength comes into its own in your weakness.'" (2 Corinthians 12:9) My Jesus is all I need…yesterday, today, and forever.

The Nightmare of the Baked Potato

Wednesday, September 12, 2012

ONCE UPON A TIME THERE was a silly little woman who had some of her body parts cut out and then was sewn back together. In spite of previous experience, the silly little woman believed that recovery should be short and easy, because, after all, she had better things to do than sit around the house and nurse her wounds. So one day, just a few weeks after the procedure, the woman made plans to meet a favorite friend for lunch. The woman planned carefully, because she knew that her body was not fully adjusted to her usual culinary delights. She thought it would be smart to meet at a casual deli where she could order a simple baked potato and her friend could enjoy the best iced tea in town. The appointed day arrived, and the woman with the scar on her belly was excited! Not only would she get to leave her house, but she was going to drive a car! And have girl talk! And wear makeup! The birds chirped happily outside her window while she lovingly bid her three small cowboys farewell. She felt a moment of sadness that they couldn't share in her big day, but alas, they had to go out into the world and conquer elementary school. The woman with the scar on her belly was finally satisfied that she looked presentable. She cheerfully drove to the restaurant and greeted her friend with a big hug. They went inside the restaurant, and the woman marveled at how light and bright everything looked. After weeks within the four walls of her own home, the outside world appeared bigger and more beautiful than ever! When it was time to order, she was tempted by the best sweet tea the town had to offer, but took the high road and stuck to her plan: a baked potato and a glass of water. Well, the two friends had a marvelous time. They laughed and swapped stories and cried, and then laughed a whole lot more. As the woman believed the simple baked potato was nourishing her broken body, the fellowship was also nourishing her soul. As she talked with her friend, the woman felt satisfied—even a little proud—that she had accomplished their little luncheon. "Take THAT, you $%&*! cancer!," she thought. The thought had just popped into her head when it was interrupted by strange noises. The noises started soft and slow, but they quickly grew louder and more intense. The woman didn't even have time to look around the restaurant before she knew that those noises were coming from her. It was her post-operative stomach, expressing its apparent distaste for the lunch the little woman had so proudly fed it. The woman with the scar on her belly suspected that her day was about to take a downhill turn. She quickly hugged her friend, promised a "next time," and jumped in her car. Thankfully, she was not too far from home, but each rumble from her stomach seemed to stretch the route. She came to a screeching halt in her driveway, and made it inside in just enough time for the baked potato to be disposed of. More than once. And then the toast she'd had for breakfast. And all of the food she had consumed in the previous days and weeks. All gone. After more than an hour, the woman lay on her empty, scarred-up belly, spent. Every part of her ached. She silently cursed the humble potato for acting

Allyson Hendrickson

so innocent when really it was setting a trap for hungry people with digestive issues. She cursed herself for foolishly believing in the potato. Suddenly, the woman heard a noise! It seemed to echo throughout the too-quiet house. Could it be…? YES! It was the sound of a door opening. And footsteps. Someone was in the house with her! Before the woman could think what to do, a pair of shoes met her at eye-level. The woman looked up and was relieved to see that the legs in those (cute) shoes belonged to her mother. She was saved! As her little mother sank to the floor next to her, the woman with the scar on her belly managed to croak, "It's not as bad as it looks." Even though it was. From that day on, the woman was terrified of food and only ate white rice. The End

What I Want

Tuesday, October 02, 2012

"You may be at odds with God right now. You're not happy with the way your life is turning out. You may be praying and pleading with God. But is it possible you don't really want God? Is it possible you just want what you think God can give you? One of the things I believe God is teaching me in my life these days is that at times we want our dreams more than we want God. We want what God does for us instead of just God."

—Pete Wilson,

Plan B: What Do You Do When God Doesn't Show Up the Way You Thought He Would?

I'M NOT HAPPY WITH THE way my life is turning out. Right now, I have cancer. I have no job. I have a car, but nowhere really to go. I have mouth sores from the chemo that have forced me to eat applesauce and oatmeal for every meal for two weeks. I have dreams that are dashed. I have a 5th grader who suddenly thinks I am the most uncool person on the planet and a 3rd grader with hurt feelings. I have someone close to me who is facing a giant mountain, and we are climbing it together. Nope, this life is not at all what I had pictured.

Yes, I pray and I plead. Lately, my prayers go something like this: "Lord, I am begging you for healing. Please take this awful disease and kick it where the sun don't shine. Please be Jehovah-Rapha, the Healer God, and prove your power through me." OR "God, why did you make tweenagers to be so ornery? Why doesn't this kid remember that I went down through the valley of the shadow of death to get him into this world? Please help him realize that I deserve his best moods and affections every day." OR "God, I can't talk to you today because my mouth hurts TOO MUCH!!! Please fix these sores so we can try again tomorrow." Amen and amen.

I want things from God. I want for God to zap the kid at school who is being unkind to my Little Middle. I want my body to be whole and healthy. I want a big fat bank account. I want a long life with my husband and a house in the country with two rocking chairs on the front porch. I want to eat hamburgers again. I want to dance with my sons at their weddings, and then be Super-Grandma when their babies come along. I want normal. I want, I want, I want…

But the Christian life isn't about my plan. It's not my way or my wants. When I accepted Christ some 30 yeas ago, I accepted his ways. I realized that things might not always go the way I wanted them to, and I said that as long as I had Jesus, I would be OK with that. Have I really gotten so caught up in what's wrong that I bypass Who is right?

The truth is, I don't want to be that shallow or that selfish. At age six, I didn't know much, but I knew that I was a sinner. I needed a Savior, and I still need Him as much today as I did then. It's time for a reality check. It's time to re-read the old promises and claim them as my own. It's time for refreshment and renewal. It's time to be still and focus on what I need. I need Jesus.

My new prayer might sound a little something like this: "Less of me, more of You, no matter what may come. I want all of You, and only You, Jesus."

Light in the Darkness

Friday, October 05, 2012

> Have I not commanded you? Be strong and courageous.
> Do not be terrified, do not be discouraged, for the Lord
> your God will be with you wherever you go. (Joshua 1:9)

THIS IS THE VERSE THAT I posted yesterday morning on Facebook as I prepared to leave for the hospital. I was up against Chemo #2, and I was feeling anything but strong and courageous. I needed the reminder that Jesus was going with me. Four hours later, I was more terrified and more discouraged than ever before. After a lengthy wait (what is it with doctors' offices, anyway?!?), I was not able to take the chemo treatment. Dr. F determined that I was still not recovered enough from #1 for my body to accept the Doxil. The stubborn and horrific mouth sores and a new skin issue were enough reason for him to pause and re-think. He decided that the dosage of chemo should be reduced, and we will try again on Tuesday. If the reduced dosage is still problematic, I may need to make a decision about continuing treatment. Talk about discouraged. Discouraged barely scrapes the surface of what my heart feels. I wrote this to a friend who is traveling her own cancer road: "…this SUCKS. I am so sick of cancer dictating everything about my life, even down to what I write on (and cross off) my calendar. I hate it that I feel like I'm free-falling and that this old world is taking huge chunks from me…my energy, my body, my family—ugh. I want so much to be a light, but the darkness is so DARK." She described back to me that I'm right (love you, H!), and she feels as if she is in a dark house, just looking for slits of light. Yeah. Just a crack here and there, Lord, would be enough to help me plant my feet. A tiny flashlight to navigate my way out of this. That's all I need. And you promised to go with me. WHERE ARE YOU?!?!? Ding-dong. I didn't move to answer the door because I was busy feeling sorry for myself, and I was sure it was just one of the neighborhood kids who seem to flock to my house every day after school. "Mommy? Somebody's here. It's for you." Standing in my entryway was an old teacher friend of mine (by old, you must know I mean "from way back," not "aged"). We feel tender toward each other, but we don't have much opportunity to run in the same circles much anymore. She said, "I don't know what's going on, but I felt like I was supposed to stop at your house and bring you dinner." Friends have faithfully been bringing food while I've been ill, but yesterday was our "off" day. It hadn't occurred to me that I needed to conjure up a meal to feed my family. I burst into tears. And just like that, the light re-appeared through the crevices of my darkness. With two carry-out pizzas and a plate of brownies, God proved—again—that He is faithful. That he is real. That he cares. That he uses ordinary people to do his work. And that I never, ever, have to feel terrified or discouraged. I may go on Tuesday and be turned away again. I may receive treatment and go back to being isolated with my crazy red skin and wretched mouth sores. I may be forced to make the terrible choice of giving up the one drug that could save my life in exchange for valuable, quality time. I don't know what my future holds, but I know who holds my future: Jesus, the Father of Light.

Allyson Hendrickson

> Suddenly, God, your light floods my path; God drives out the darkness. (2 Samuel 22:29)

P.S. Because I couldn't have chemo, I could go to a high school football game with my trio of cowboys. How 'bout this guy?

Doxil 2/6

Tuesday, October 16, 2012

I WANT TO PREFACE THIS post by saying that I take back everything nice I said about Doxil before. So there. I was originally scheduled to have my second Doxil treatment on Thursday, October 4. The pre-treatment visit with Dr. F made it clear that the staff would be unable to administer chemo that day due to mouth sores and a crazy skin thing, both caused by the Doxil itself. It seems a little weird to me that the drug is responsible for these outrageous side effects, but the side effects have to be completely cleared up in order for me to safely accept the drug. Whatever. I left the hospital more than a little discouraged, armed with instructions to come back the following Tuesday so we could "try again." Mom and I followed directions and were there before the appointed time on Tuesday the 9th. This time I passed inspection and we were sent down to the chemo room. We immediately picked up on an invisible power struggle going on between the two chemo nurses. One definitely seems much more competent and patient-friendly than the other (to me, anyway), but does it really matter whose side of the room has more heating pads? I felt especially sorry for Keith, the new guy, whose job it is to collect patients' vital signs, document medications, and otherwise be at the nurses' beck and call while learning the ropes. I had some apprehension about my port. The last time I had treatment, I had just come straight from surgery and the surgeon had just left the port accessed for chemo. Today I would find out what "accessing the port" really means. Bottom line: IT HURTS. As I write this one week later, the area around the port is still tender and sore. I would much prefer to have IV lines started each time. I fail to see what the big advantage is! My pre-meds went down with no problems. Just when I was getting comfy with my pink hoodie and my zebra blanket, the nurse had a new fun surprise. She started the Doxil, and then she brought over two huge ice packs. One went on the floor and I was made to rest my feet on top of it; the other was for my hands. Additionally, I was given a cup of crushed ice. The presumption is that ice slows the circulation of blood to the extremities during treatment, which in turn lessens the chances of sores popping up in the weeks after. I am in favor, of course, of avoiding painful sores on my hands and feet and inside my mouth, but I was freezing. I had to keep the ice on me the entire hour that it took for the Doxil bag to drip. It seems hard to believe that in the year 2012, we don't have any more sophisticated method of preventing chemo-related sores! We made it home with plenty of time to spare before the cowboys got home from school. I went straight to bed, not feeling terrible, but not feeling great, either. And so it has gone for most of the last week. While I have had some bouts of nausea, I haven't felt terribly sick. Mostly, I feel tired. Fatigued. Exhausted. I can be working my way through a day, and suddenly I just have the overwhelming urge to lie down. That usually results in a "nap" that lasts 3–4 hours! These naps have been defined by nonsensically vivid dreams. One day I dreamt that I lived in a 2-bedroom apartment in the ghetto. My friend Rachel, aka Moldy, brought over a random baby boy for me to take care of, but he was dressed in girl clothes. My neighbor loaned me her double stroller for this babysitting bout, which was chrome and outfitted in the latest "hooptie" styles. Another neighbor insisted that I join her in a field and fly kites with her because we were running out of wind energy. Strange. Another dream had me dressed up in Little House on the Prairie-ish clothes, running through an old Indian village. As I ran in and out of teepees I shouted, "Sanctuary! Sanctuary!" I finally found safety in a nearby saloon, only to be discovered by a little boy I used to teach who I suppose grew up to be a bad guy. A dream over the weekend involved a wartime airplane. I was decked out in goggles and a scarf, and I expertly landed my plane in the desert. I had nothing to eat but cactus, which was lucky because somehow I knew how to cut a cactus just right so as to get the grape jelly out of it. People I went to high school with were there, but their cacti did not have any grape jelly. I guess they weren't properly trained. So, one week in to the 2nd cycle, I am tired. The good news is that I seem to have finally turned a corner with my new and not-so-large intestine. I am still very cautious with what I eat, but I have been pleasantly surprised to find that I am finally able to eat some meat, a few finely-chopped fruits and veggies, and even one slice of pizza the other day! I still have not worked up the courage to test another baked potato, though. It will be a while before I feel that brave. I continue to ask God for protection from illness, germs, and sores. I thank Him when I wake up and realize that I am not really Laura Ingalls or Amelia Earheart, and that I have enough sense to find those crazy sleep scenarios comical. I am glad when I stay up later than my kids, and I am thankful when my Hubby sends me to bed, even if it is a ridiculously early time. I plead with God that Doxil, with all of its quirks, would be THE drug that I need it to be. I know that so many friends, family, and even strangers are pleading with me and for me. Thank you. He is good, and He does good.

Heaven Is Only a Dream Away

Tuesday, November 27, 2012

I HAD A DREAM. My dream was intense and very realistic. Most importantly, it has brought me peace. In my dream… I went to heaven. When I got there, there was no huge gate with Saint Peter sitting behind a big desk. There were no angels with wings floating around. When I got there, there was only one person: my Grandad. He was waiting for me. He knew I was coming. He looked exactly the same as he did most of my life: he was strong with big hands, a big smile, and very little hair. He was wearing his standard "uniform": a golf shirt and slacks. Only, in heaven, his shirt was white. Bright white, like Gran had washed it with Clorox. As soon as Grandad saw me, he smile grew wide and he said, "I've been waiting for you, girl. Come on in." He put his strong arm around me and we walked into heaven. Grandad took me into a section that looked like a suburban neighborhood with big, beautiful houses on both sides of the street. The street was white with a fog rising up off of it, almost like someone had a dry ice machine. Where there might have been yards in front of each house, there was instead shimmery white light—sort of like a tub full of bubbles. There were no trees, no grass, but it was very, very beautiful. There were no other beings in sight, or even signs of life. The only movement was from me and my Grandad, walking side by side. Finally he stopped in front of the biggest house. He said, "This is it. I want to show you around." I wasn't sure at all what to expect, but I was not afraid. He opened the door, and I immediately felt warmth and coziness. It was the feeling of home. I get a similar feeling when I sit in front of our Christmas tree, loving the lights. Or after the boys go to bed and the house is still and quiet. It is a feeling of contentment and belonging. We stepped in to the house. Grandad said, "I've been getting things ready for you." Before I explain what he meant, I should let you know a little something about my Grandad. When he lived here on earth, he was a builder. Not for his job, but after he retired, he spent a lot of time here: He made treasure boxes and bookshelves and tea trays. All of us have some precious keepsake in our homes that was fashioned by Grandad's hands. So it really was no surprise in heaven that Grandad had a workshop. It looked just like his red-roof shop that stands silently now, except that the roof, the walls, even the sign—were white. Grandad had been working hard. His restored body had added on to the place that God had ready for him when he left us in 2008. As he walked me through the home, he proudly showed me each room. Each was large, and the furniture was gleaming white. There were rooms for each member of our family. God and Grandad had made sure that our family would be together for eternity. Each aunt and uncle had a room. Every cousin (plus their significant other and their children) had a space of their own. There was a room for Buck and Grandmama, my other grandparents. In his own room, Grandad showed me the "pretty things" that he knew Gran would love. There was a table covered in white porcelain figurines and tea cups—girly trinkets, if you will. He was ready for her to join him.

The last room was mine. Grandad pushed open the door, and I entered in amazement. The room was cavernous. There was a toolbox (white, of course) on the floor that looked just like the one Hubby's Papa gave him. Grandad picked it up quickly and explained that he had been making some last-minute adjustments because he knew I was coming. I remember that the rooms had beds, but the unspoken understanding was that they would never need to be used for sleeping or nursing a sickness, in the sense that I use my bed now. They were simply for comfort. There was space in my room for Hubby and my little cowboys. Grandad knew they would be coming later. I was not fearful or sad to be separated from them. I, too, knew that they were coming. After the house tour was over, Grandad led me back out the front door. The house had a massive front porch with white railings, much like the one I've "pinned" onto my "Dreams" board on Pinterest. Grandad had built two Cracker Barrel-like rocking chairs. He sat in one, I sat in the other. He took my hand in his, and we began to rock back and forth in perfect rhythm. My grandfather said, "Now, girl, all we have to do is wait for the others." I woke up with a smile on my face. It was more than a dream to me…it was an experience. I felt—and still feel—an intense peace that I haven't known for as long as I've had The Sickness. I don't know what the outcome of The Sickness will be, but I am certain that ultimately, my dream will become my reality. This old body betrays me. But when it gives out, I WILL GO HOME. And what a glorious home is waiting for me!

When I Am Afraid...

Thursday, December 06, 2012

Doxil 3/6 has not been fun. Or easy. Or calm. Or without drama. Last week, I had mouth sores that reduced me to using a dry-erase white board to communicate with my family. Luckily, the cowboys thought that was a great game! I also had the skin affliction in full swing, meaning that standing under a shower felt like being pelted with bullets. My yoga pants were the only fabric that could comfortably touch me, and big chunks of skin were peeling off of my feet and toes. Horrible, stupid side effects. The other thing I had last week was appointments. After 3 treatments, I am at the halfway point with chemo. I had an appointment to have an echocardiogram done to check for any damage that Doxil may be doing to my heart. I also had an appointment for a CT scan, which would provide a picture for my medical team to look for complications, and ultimately, recurrent cancer.

The echo came back clear. My heart is still pumping perfectly. The scan, however, was a different story. The radiologist who read the scan saw spots that have the appearance of recurrent carcinomas. This news was delivered to me by a solemn-faced Dr. F. I could tell that he was concerned. Frankly, I think that he has a terrible job. Why anyone would want to be an oncologist (or a dentist) is beyond me. Anyway, there was a decision to be made. I could assume that the spots are scar tissue (or some other medical thing that I don't understand) and carry on with the Doxil treatments as planned. OR I could take a more proactive approach and have a biopsy done. Although the idea of yet another procedure was less than appealing, I feel strongly that I have to know what I'm up against. If I have cancer growing in my body in spite of active chemo treatment, I have a bigger problem than I thought and I need to make big decisions. The implications of that scenario are overwhelming. If it is not cancer, I can breathe a little easier and keep fighting. I opted for the biopsy. The procedure, although uncomfortable, went fine. I was told that my doctor's office would contact me with results. As of this morning, the results are still not in. So I wait. Waiting is really, really hard. It means that I have a lot of time on my hands and I have to fill it, or else I'll go crazy. I went to a spelling bee (Goliath won his class bee, then placed 5th in the school bee. Proud mom!). I went Christmas shopping with my mom. I'm catching up on some reading and some crafting. I've done FaceTime with Reese the Niece. I'm taking Little Middle to the dentist tomorrow (although he doesn't know it yet).

And through all of that, I pretend that I am a normal girl with an "normal" life. Just looking at me, you wouldn't know that I'm desperately afraid, and that my entire life hinges on a phone call that has yet to come. "When I am afraid, I will put my trust in You." Psalm 56:3 Trusting God means that I believe that He has the best for me. Always. No matter what. I don't see how cancer can be the best thing for me, or for the people I love. I can't fathom how this blow is to my benefit. I'm not sure how to not waiver while waiting. But I want to trust. I DO trust. Lord, I am scared. I am tired. I am uncertain. But I love you and I know that you are good. My hope is in you alone.

Close

Friday, December 07, 2012

Goliath's jiu jitsu class is a great place for me to talk on the phone. I am stuck there for a solid 45 minutes while he punches and wrestles his little heart out, which is plenty of time to play catch up. This was the case yesterday. I spent a good 25 minutes chatting and sharing with a long-time friend. We had just hung up when my phone rang again. The caller ID said that the caller was "unknown." In my world, that means it's the oncology office.

It was Dr. F. I'm not sure that he has ever called me himself before. Isn't that why doctors have minions? To do the bothersome work of communicating and scheduling? But this news was far too important to assign to a minion to deliver. I knew it as soon as I heard his voice.

The news is bad. New cancer is growing in my body. It is growing out of nothing, at the same time that active poison chemotherapy is being delivered into my body.

We were both silent for a moment. Neither of us knew what to say. Then I took a deep breath, tuned out the sounds of punching bags around me, and said the only thing I could think of: "Well, this really sucks." He agreed.

The course of action is up to me. Obviously, I am done with Doxil. Dr. F assured me that the problem is not necessarily that the Doxil wasn't working. The real problem we face is that the cancer that plagues me is big and fast and aggressive and strong. It simply overpowered the drug. So, I am going straight to the next drug. Remember when I told you that Doxil was the one and only possibility? That list is still true, but in my case will serve as more of a guideline than an end-all cancer Bible. I've given the go-ahead for the medical team to stuff Doxil and move on to topotecan. It is standard, as far as chemotherapy goes. I will be nauseous and sick. I will be very susceptible to infection due to low blood cell counts, and weak. I will possibly lose my hair. The plan now is to do six cycles. One cycle means treatment once a week for three weeks, with the fourth week off. I will start immediately.

The reason that I have to do this is simple, and can be divided into three parts: Goliath, Little Middle, and Baby. I may not be the best mother in the world, but I am their mother. Made for them. I'm the only one they are ever going to get. I will not—WILL NOT!!—do anything less than everything for my sons. This disease may kill me, but not without a hard fight.

Last night I cried with my husband and my mother. I called my dad, my sister, and my brother and cried again. The sorrow among the six of us is overwhelming. The despair, the anger, the absolute grief—too much. The hurt…oh, the hurt! I think our hearts must be broken, but none of us have the luxury of giving in to heartbreak. Because there are three little cowboys who need their mom.

I am close to the edge. I'm teetering on the side of keeping it together. I am so close that I can look over into the pit of despair and hopelessness. If I am pushed ever so slightly…if I get one more phone call…if I have to make one more decision…if one more inkling of uncertainty darkens my doorstep…I could just give in and let go. I could surrender to the inclination to cover my head and hide out until I die. And who would blame me?

But there are these little men who call me "Mom." And some days, when I'm really lucky, I still get to be "Mommy." And I have this God who I sure don't understand, but he promises to stay close to me because I am brokenhearted and my spirit is crushed (Psalm 34:18). I know that I am not done. I'm close, but I can back up, take a deep breath, dry my tears, and look ahead. Brokenhearted, but not beaten.

The Night before Chemo

Monday, December 10, 2012

'Twas the night before chemo, when all through the house,
were my kids and my mother and Hubby, my spouse. School lunches were packed by the Nana with care
As I dragged boys to bed up every last stair.

The cowboys were nestled snug in their beds,
With lyrics of Christmas songs stuck in their heads.
And Mom in her pjs and me in the same Both were worn out from the $%&! cancer game.

When up in my head
there arose such a clatter
I sat up in bed
to think what was the matter.
Away to my blog
I flew like a flash,
Opened my laptop
Praying it wouldn't crash.

The gleam on the screen of my trusty old Dell
gave me a chance for my story to tell.

Three Little Cowboys

When, what to my wandering mind did I think
I should make an appointment to go see a shrink!

More rapid than eagles the images came,
And I got mad, and shouted, and called them by name:
"Dumb sickness! Dumb chemo! I hate you a lot!
Mean nurses! Cold tubing! My blood will not clot!
Stop touching my port! Stop giving me meds!
Now dash away! dash away! or off with your heads!"

And then in a twinkling
I knew in my mind
That sure enough, I was in a big bind.
I reigned in my thoughts and settled on down,
Then something else happened that caused me to frown.

My hair was two colors, and getting quite thin,
And my clothes were too scratchy for my sensitive skin.
My stomach was rumbling from the inside out
And I felt like I needed a drink that was stout.

My eyes used to twinkle
But now they're ablaze
And my soul is determined to fight through these days.
When the morning comes and I rise from my bed
I surely know I have nothing to dread.

I spoke not a word, but bowed my head to pray.
"Lord, give me the strength I need for that day."
Then, knowing that my God was holding me tight,
I reached to the lamp and turned off the light.

A Letter to My Sons

Tuesday, December 18, 2012

DEAR GOLIATH, LITTLE MIDDLE, AND Baby, Something big happened on Friday, December 14. It didn't happen here. It didn't happen to us. But it was big just the same, and I can't—and don't want to—just shake it off and get on with life as usual. I didn't want to tell you that a sad, sick person went into an elementary school. It was a school just like the one the three of you go to every day. I didn't want you to know that he had weapons and an intent to kill, that he wanted to cause harm to children who are just like you. I wanted to protect you from knowing that the world can be such a scary, awful place. But I couldn't. You are each so smart, and there was no hiding from you the rampant news coverage, the solemn moods of the adults around you, and the half-mast flags that are all over town. You asked all the right questions, if there even is such a thing as "right" in this horrible situation. You wanted to know what happened, and if it could happen to you, too. You asked about the children and the teachers. How did the bad man get in? How did he kill them? How did they get out? And you asked the question that most of our country is asking: WHY? Oh, little loves. Why, indeed? We, of course, have talked a lot in our house about why God allows bad things to happen to good people. Although I don't necessarily like it, I've thought that maybe, in terms of my cancer and our other family heartache, that I might have figured it out. I've told you that if I—if WE—trust God and we are faithful to Him, than our suffering is not in vain. He promises good things because we love Him. He promises to take care of all of us and to give us exactly what we need.

But my suffering is easier for me to process because I am a grown up. I've had a life full of experiences and mistakes, happiness and sorrow, growing and learning. I never say it out loud to you, but I think you already know that you, my babies, are the reasons I worry so much AND why I fight to get well. Because you have everything ahead of you. I don't want you to be frightened or worried or disadvantaged or helpless. Most mommies want the best for their children, just like I do for you.

Those children in Newtown had everything ahead of them. Their mommies helped them get dressed on Friday morning. Maybe they rushed them through breakfast the way I sometimes do. Maybe some of them sang silly songs about the weather, or maybe some of them had to ask more than once if teeth had been brushed and hair combed. Some of those mommies might have been flustered or annoyed, or maybe they loved mornings that bring the promise of a new day. Some might have even been relieved when they dropped their kids off and came home to a quiet house. I have mornings like that.

I don't know why. As much as I want to assure you that you are safe, I know that would be dishonest. Daddy and I do our best, but this world is so broken, sweet sons. There is so much hurt and people are damaged in millions of ways. You, maybe better than a lot of other kids, know what real suffering is. I'm sorry that I can't protect you like I want to. I'm sorry that you will remember December 14, 2012 as a day that you felt scared. Will you do this for me? Let's try to remember December 14, 2012 as a day that

Allyson Hendrickson

we were reminded of what we already know is true: God loves you. God cares about you, down to the smallest detail. God is with you everywhere you go. The Bible is absolutely true. God wants good things for you.

God gave you to me, the three greatest gifts of my lifetime. You are mine only for a time, though, because He and I both know that you really belong to Him. I promise you that I will hug you a little tighter in the mornings. I will listen a little more intently when you talk, I will soak up every minute I get to spend with you, and I will look for every opportunity to teach you Truth. Your Daddy and I love you with everything that we have and we are. So do your Poppy and Nana and your Papa and Mema. But nobody—not even me—loves you the way that God loves you. Love people without reserve, show kindness and respect to everyone, and live large, boys. The world can be scary, but you can be and do anything. YOU ARE LOVED.

With my whole heart, Mom

Mack

Sunday, December 23, 2012

So, chemo's not going so well. Actually, I think that chemo is going exactly as it is supposed to. I do this funny thing where I just decide that things are going to happen a certain way. I seem to think that just by sheer willpower I can escape side effects that are universal with chemotherapy. Silly, huh? I set myself up for disappointment when I actually sleep for three days, or when I stand in front of the refrigerator wondering why we don't have anything good to eat.

So the universe will have to forgive me for not feeling as Christmassy as I ought to. Yes, all of my gifts are purchased and wrapped. The tree is still standing straight (usually by this time it's leaning to one side or the other). I've caroled, shopped, churched, baked, and traditioned myself as much as possible. One might say I'm ready for Christmas. But I know the truth. I have been too tired and honestly, feeling a little too sorry for myself to get into the spirit.

This morning I woke up determined to do something beyond the four walls of my bedroom, where I've been since my last infusion on Tuesday. I wanted to bake cookies. There are certain tastes and smells that mean "Christmas," and I wanted them in my house today. So I went to Wal-Mart. I needed only a few things—powdered sugar, butter, eggs. I didn't bother much with makeup or wardrobe. I just wanted to go fast so I could get home fast.

I was so caught up in hiding my non-made-up face behind my big sunglasses that I didn't notice him at first. I was in a rush, but Mack was not. He never is. Mack is a greeter at my local Wally World. It's his job to say hello to everyone, give directions, wipe down shopping carts, and put stickers on return items. If I had to guess, I'd peg him in his mid-sixties but it wouldn't surprise me if he was younger. He walks with a limp, as if he never quite healed from an old injury.

Now, I'm more of a Kroger girl when it comes to grocery shopping, but there are days (like today) that the Mart is good for one-stop shopping. I've been there enough to know that Mack is a fixture. He is as steady as the stream of people that pass by him each day. He stands in the entryway of the giant store, often leaning on a cart to support his weak leg. He must get tired. He has to be bored. I can't imagine spending hours every day at such a menial task. Better Mack than me.

But this morning, the Saturday before Christmas, when I was completely wrapped up in ME, Mack made a difference. He greeted me, like he's done a hundred times before. There were people in front of me, and lots of people behind me. But Mack made me feel like I was the only person there. He gave me a huge smile that showed his teeth, made eye contact with me, and then he said, "Merry Christmas."

And as I pushed my cart into the aisles with all the other Saturday-before-Christmas crazies, I couldn't help but think: Mack gets Christmas. Mack IS Christmas. Mack works a seemingly unimportant job that surely doesn't pay nearly enough. He is physically inept. From where I (and most of you) stand, he is at some disadvantage. But Mack embodies the spirit of this season: J-O-Y. He made me believe in our second of contact that there was nowhere else he would rather be than right there in that windy atrium, welcoming me to my friendly neighborhood Wal-Mart. He made me think that I mattered, and he had the smile and the kindness to back it up. He put someone else ahead of his own needs and wants.

That sounds like quite a load to attribute to a man I don't even know, doesn't it? Maybe so. But when it is so easy to get lost in the endless to-do lists, and when the budget it blown, and when "peace on earth" is out of sight, and when the season doesn't make sense…I think we should be even more on the lookout for the true spirit of Christmas. So here's to you, Mack…have yourself a merry little Christmas. As for me, I baked those little almond cookies and sprinkled them liberally with sugar. Tonight I will share them with my family and make a new holiday memory. 'Tis the season.

I Think That If I Get My Hair Cut, It Won't Be So Long.

Thursday, January 10, 2013

Round Two began this week. Going back to chemo after having last week off was super-hard. I had a week of driving the little cowboys to and fro about the town. I did a lot of cooking for my little family. I played with my boys, ran errands, and even did my own grocery shopping! "Normal" has never felt so nice.

But, as it always does, Tuesday came around again. First up was a visit with Bruce himself, the almighty Dr. F. My mom thinks that Dr. F greatly resembles Stephen Colbert, even to the point that she wonders what my oncologist is doing on television some nights. Anyway…my time with Dr. F can be summarized with a quick game of "I Said, He Said." Here it goes:

I said… He said nausea… crackers hair… wig headaches… MRI ouch!… sorry Sugar Land…Thai food Round One of Topotecan has come and gone, leaving plenty of misery in its wake. The nausea and sickness factor can best be described as similar to morning sickness during pregnancy. While I'm not throwing up, the feeling of being ill never quite lifts. I feel hungry, but no food looks or sounds good. I need to be drinking gallons of water to prevent dehydration, but small sips throughout the day seem to be all that I can muster. Do you know how much energy it takes to reach over and pick up a cup of water?!? More than I can spare. Energy is a premium resource these days. It must be preserved at all costs because it is in such short supply. My head aches. I have noticed that headaches have become more frequent and more severe in the last several weeks. Most mornings I wake up with one, and I have been taking alarming amounts of pain killers to stave them off. Mentioning it to Dr. F seemed like the right thing to do, but it earned me a same-day appointment at the imaging center across the street for a MRI. Unbelievably, I have never had an MRI before. I would remember wearing a hockey mask in a coffin while a jackhammer is pounding in my ears. I am seriously questioning which is worse: the MRI or my known nemesis, the CT scan? The MRI results were fine. There is no cancer growing in my brain (thank God!). There is, however, a malformation that the test detected that is known as a chiari one. Basically, it means that my skull did not grow big enough to accommodate my brain. Pressure build-up occurs, which can be the cause of the headaches I am experiencing. As a precaution, I will be seeing a neurologist soon to discuss treatment. Until then, I am reveling in the I-told-you-so rights this news earned me. I've spent years telling my brother how smart I am!

About my hair…I knew going in to this treatment that hair loss was a possibility. Unlike the Taxol regimen I did a couple of years ago, hair loss with Topotecan is not 100%. Most materials refer to the hair loss as "thinning," with a few unlucky patients going completely bald. Honestly, I wasn't too worried about it… until I started noticing that my hair was everywhere. Over the last two weeks, I have plucked zillions of hairs out of my sweaters and off of my shoulders. I have swept them off the floor, brushed them off of my pillowcase, and rescued massive amounts from going down the drain in the shower. Morning styling results in a mini-shower of hair raining down around me. I had to do something.

In discussing this predicament with my mother, I mentioned that I probably ought to make a trip to the hairdresser, because "I think that if I get my hair cut, it won't be so long." Yep. That's a gem.

So that's what I did. My hair, which has not been touched by professional hands since my re-diagnosis last summer, has now been chopped off and coaxed to look like that of a healthy person. Only I know that it is in such a fragile state, that if you look at it wrong, it might wilt right off of my head. Dr. F kindly suggested that I pull out my old Taxol-era wigs, so I can be ready just in case. The pretend hair is on stand-by.

If I think about it for any length of time, I am stunned—absolutely STUNNED—that this is my life. This sick-looking, hair-thinning, sleep-round-the-clock girl is ME. The face staring back at me in the mirror loves her children more than life itself. She wants to eat Blue Bell for breakfast, read a book on a park bench, and travel 'round the world, but she's not doing any of it. Because she has cancer. Most days, I take it in stride because, well, I have to. But some days, like today, when I cut my hair because it's falling out, all I can feel is dismay. And fear. And I wonder what ever happened to the old Allyson…and will she ever be back?

Hair and Heartache

Sunday, February 10, 2013

EVERY SINGLE MORNING, NO MATTER how sick I feel, I get up and sit with my little cowboys while they have breakfast and get ready for their day. I want them to understand that they matter more to me than anything that I have going on, including The Sickness. It was not unusual, then, that I sat at the table yesterday with Goliath and Little Middle. I looked a hot mess, after 3 days of a chemo-induced semi-coma. The boys were thrilled to start their Saturday off with bowls of Cinnamon Toast Crunch and some Mom time. At least, until they heard what I had to say. It had to do with my hair. How it is falling out—"thinning" is the term from the oncology literature—and has been for some time now. How I think it's time to do something, but I don't want them to be embarrassed or have to explain to their friends…And before the rest of the thought could make its way out of my mouth, my sweet boys jumped right in: "You can wear your wig when you go to church or to our school!" "I know where your scarves and hats are upstairs. Do you want me to go get them?" "I'm not embarrassed. If anyone asks why you don't have any hair, I'll just tell them it's because you have cancer and they better mind their own business!" (This from my fiercely-protective Goliath, with his eyes flashing—I dare anyone to cross him.) And…"Mom, we think you're pretty."

Oh, my darling boys. I could barely keep the tears in while I hugged them, reminded them to put their cereal bowls in the dishwasher, and fled to the safety of my bedroom.

My bedroom, with its soft gray walls and pretty blue bedding and pictures of happier days gone by, is where I feel safe. Right now, that's my haven. It's where I stay when I'm sick; it's where I go when I'm scared. "Scared" is a feeling I am well acquainted with. It goes along with "overwhelmed" and "lost." The thing with my hair isn't really new; in fact, it's kind of the last straw. It's been the thing that just this week has made me think, "Well. Maybe I really should just hole up here." It's been the latest and scariest thing that makes me want to run and pull the pretty blue covers up over my head. Because in my world, there's all this other stuff…

The pages of my journal are filling up, in spite of myself. Night after night, I write. And I write and I write. How can one person who doesn't even go out much have so much to write about? That Other Heartache drags on, albeit in a lesser form. There is so much fear wrapped up in it, and it has a powerful grip on me. Drama. And a tremendous sense of responsibility for other people's well-being and happiness. Oh. My. Goodness. Achieving and maintaining healthy relationships is exhausting work. I asked Dr. F about a long-term prognosis. It isn't pretty. And you'd think that if you KNOW that you have a limited time to live, that you would proceed like Tim McGraw's "Live Like You Were Dyin'." Only I think that for now, this chemo is the right thing to do, and it might give me more time. But it also keeps me from yanking my kids out of school so we can all jump out of an airplane together. I can't win. A funny thing about being chronically ill is that you lose your sense of belonging. My life is now measured in treatments and doctor visits, while the rest of the world carries on just as it did before The Sickness. I don't know why it surprises me so much that my friends, my Bible Study class, group...whoever! can function without me. But they remain stunned.

This life of mine, it's heavy. And right now, it's really, re... It is every moment feeling dragged under, held down, gasp breath after breath after breath. It is Dory encouraging to "just keep swimming, just keep swimming," only it isn't fu at all. It is pictures of what used to be or thoughts of wha to come that flash through my head on a never-ending reel, constant reminder that with or without me, they'll go on. It is the relentless cycle of sunrise to sunset. I dread the dawning of a new day simply because the number of hours it brings to be conquered are overwhelming. How does one start putting one foot in front of the other when she is already so far behind?

> But I pray to you, O Lord, in the time of your favor; in your great love, O God, answer me with your sure salvation. Rescue me from the mire, do not let me sink; deliver me from those who hate me, from the deep waters. Do not let the floodwaters engulf me or the depths swallow me up or the pit close its mouth over me. Answer me, O Lord, out of the goodness of your love; in your great mercy turn to me. Do not hide your face from your servant; answer me quickly, for I am in trouble. Come near and rescue me. (Psalm 69:13–18)

Not Alone

Saturday, February 23, 2013

I AM CLOSING THE BOOKS on another week, yet again feeling quite fine to see it saunter its way out. This week—oh, this week. This was the third week of the third round of the Topotecan chemotherapy cycle. All that really means is that the dreaded scan is drawing dangerously near. Next Monday, to be exact. February 25th. Yep, that's the big one. The day when one scan will supposedly give me answers to all of my biggest questions: Is the chemo working? Is the cancer growing? Am I dying? My anxiety grows with every passing hour.

That sounds dramatic, but it's really true. However, let's back up. I had the pleasure of my daddy accompanying me to chemo this week. While I would never use the word "fun" to describe such an adventure, I don't mind telling you that it made me giggle a few times to point out the staff (who I refer to as the "cast of characters") and to gauge his reactions to things that have become old hat to me. Especially when Q-Tip Tammy (an infusion nurse who resembles a human Q-Tip) raced by, cackling all the way. She's something.

But, as it always does, chemotherapy worked its dark magic and tossed me into the sea of sickness. I don't know why some weeks are more, well, blah than others, but this was one of those weeks. The nausea was definitely more intense. The temptation to cover my head and hide was stronger. We had a thunderstorm on Wednesday morning, and I was actually angry that it didn't last longer. How DARE God not let it rain 24 hours a day while I was feeling so…RAINY?!? And then the sun came out. The nerve!

I don't know if it is possible to describe what it feels like to be plunged—over and over again—into that sea. For several days after my treatment, I sleep. I lose most of my sense of time, depending on the alarm on my phone (which Goliath got hold of and changed to bark like a dog—how annoying is that?) to wake me up when the morning comes 'round so I can see my boys off to school. A quick shower and fresh pj's, and all of my energy is used up. That's it. I go back to bed, and depend on my mom to fill in for me.

That's why it sliced a little deeper when the school nurse called on Thursday with a sick Little Middle in her office. Yes, he had complained of a sore throat that morning, and yes, I had given him 2 Advil and sent him to school anyway. No Mom-Of-The-Year Award for me. Mom went to get him, took him to the pediatrician, and walked out with a positive strep diagnosis, prescriptions for antibiotics, and strict instructions for him to "stay away from your mommy because your germs can make her really, really sick."

They had no sooner made it back to the house than the school nurse called again, this time with Goliath in her office. He had fallen and hit his head on the playground, she said, and he was behaving strangely. If it was her child, she would want him to be close by and would probably get him checked out. "Strange behavior? He's 11. That's what this kid thrives on." Those were my thoughts, but I dutifully summoned my poor mother to make yet another run to the elementary school.

Turns out that "strange behavior" is dizziness, confusion, and affected speech among other things. In the last 48 hours Goliath has seen the doctor twice and done both a CT and MRI scan. Both scans came back normal. The symptoms persist, though, and while thankfully we can rule out serious brain injury, we face some unknowns.

At the pediatrician's office yesterday morning, Goliath was sitting on the table when Dr. B came in. Dr. B did Goliath's baby well checks for the first year of his life. While she was talking about outpatient MRI vs. hospital admitting, I could clearly see in my mind's eye my baby boy, totally loving me, needing me, wanting me to take care of him. That baby boy may have morphed into a giant over these years, but some things haven't changed. In the middle of all these physical trials, with me constantly fighting the temptation to dive for shelter under my covers, there has been a sweet and welcome point of relief. Every single day this week, even if only for a few minutes, I have been reminded in a very real and tangible way that I am not walking this crazy and scary road alone. I knew it when I had a mini-meltdown with my Tuesday-turned-Monday sisters and they rallied behind me over enchiladas. I knew it when that rally cry extended to our men. I've known it nearly every day for the last 10 days when the World's Grouchiest Mailman pulled in and delivered a card from a sorority sister or classmate from HSU. The WGM doesn't know it, but his furrowed eyebrows only make it that much sweeter for me to pluck those cards from among the bills and junk mail. I knew it last night when we opened the door and there were three goody bags on our doorstep with cards that read "Get Well Goliath," "Get Well Little Middle" and "Stay Well Baby." I've known I am not alone every time my phone dings (or barks) with a text message that reminds me that someone is thinking of me and cares. I knew it when I got a for-real offer from a friend who really gets it to shave our heads together in a united effort to show the $%#&@ cancer who's in charge...and then go get a pedicure. I knew it when I received a "Sunshine Basket" from my friend Jaimie (filled with all things yellow), and a gift bag from Jana filled with things that, by her own admission, are "frivolous." I know it with each yellow prayer gram I receive from a church I've never attended, written by a person who knows me only as a name on a list. But that person believes on my behalf, and they go faithfully to pray. That is powerful, is it not?

The heartache remains. The dog is very old. Bills must be paid. The kids are sick. The cancer is there. Monday is coming. Decisions must be made. The fear can be paralyzing, if I let it. I can listen to the lies. Or I can swim. It's against the current. It's hard. And I will get tired. But I know that I am not in this alone. And in these few moments, that means everything.

"Praise be to the God and Father of our Lord Jesus Christ, the Father of compassion, and the God of all comfort, who comforts us in all our troubles, so that we can comfort those in any trouble with the comfort we ourselves receive from God." 2 Corinthians 1:3–4

Three Month Results

Tuesday, February 26, 2013

Last night I had one of those dreams that seemed so real that when I woke up it took me a minute to realize that none of it had really happened. I dreamed that I went to the Ballpark in Arlington to audition to sing the national anthem at a Rangers game. The audition actually took place AT a game in front of a sold-out crowd. I went out to the pitcher's mound, and then I forgot the words to The Star Spangled Banner. But I didn't hesitate…I sang Amazing Grace instead. A natural choice. And somehow, it was phenomenal. The crowd went wild. Ron Washington had tears in his eyes. People were throwing their hats in the air and cheering! The Rangers ran onto the field and offered me an exclusive contract to travel with them and sing Amazing Grace at every game. I was just about to sign the papers when my phone rang. I answered it. It was Dr. F. He said, "We got the scan results. I don't know how this has happened, but there has been a huge mix-up and it turns out you never had cancer to begin with." I said, "That's great, because I'm going on tour with the Texas Rangers!" and I hung up on him.

Three Little Cowboys

I've never hated my alarm clock more. Unfortunately, the Texas Rangers did not call me today. But Nurse Allyson did. At 4:30 p.m. It was a really long day. The news is not the best, nor is it the worst. The CT images show that the cancer is stable. It is basically unchanged since the last scan I had in November. Since I began the Topotecan regimen, the diseased areas have neither shrunk or grown. The cancer remains in my abdomen, just as it was three months ago. I do not know how I should feel about this news. I know it could be worse, so I feel, I don't know…guilty? that I am upset. What bothers me most, I think, is the idea of the wasted time. For three months I have gone back and forth. Three months I have spent the majority of my time sick or sleeping or incapacitated or unavailable. Three months I have been around my boys, but not with my boys. Three months. That might not seem like such a long time when you are thirty-seven. But three months to a seven-year-old boy? That's a good chunk. So…the inevitable question: What Next? Dr. F wants to order a PET scan to check on the metabolic activity of the existing cancer. This will answer a few questions (hopefully) about how the chemotherapy has affected it so that we can make an informed decision about further treatment. I will meet with the good doctor next Tuesday, March 5. Tonight, my brain is a mess of swirling thoughts and questions. I wish I could understand. I wish I could see the big picture. I wish I could look into the future and see my little boys all grown up to be men and know what the purpose is for the suffering they must endure. My confusion and fear are real, but so is my faith. I believe that my God is good, and that His love for me stretches beyond what I can comprehend.

> "Have courage for the great sorrows of life and patience for the small ones. When you have finished your daily task, go to sleep in peace. God is awake."
>
> —Victor Hugo

Unchanging

Tuesday, March 05, 2013

"The Lord is good to those whose hope is in him, to the one who seeks him." Lamentations 3:25

I went to the hospital today not knowing what to expect, so I prepared for every contingency. I half expected to meet with Dr. F and hear that the chemo was not working so I should go home. I was ready to hear that the chemo had at least stabilized the cancer, so I packed my usual chemo gear (soft blanket, purple socks, Seinfeld DVD, phone charger) in case it went on as scheduled. I made sure that Mom was ready to take notes and that Hubby had his questions waiting.

There is no way I could have been prepared for what happened in today's appointment." A faith and knowledge resting on the hope of eternal life, which God, who does not lie, promised before the beginning of time." Titus 1:2A solemn Dr. F waved a handful of papers in my general direction, but neither of us bothered to read them. We both already knew that they contained the discouraging news of the unchanging cancer in my body. The cancer that stubbornly remains, refusing to be affected by any poison or toxin, and defiantly growing back when temporarily removed.

The cancer that, it seems, is there to stay.

With gentle words and tears in his eyes, the good doctor recommended that I return to MD Anderson as soon as possible. Sweet Nurse Allyson had already begun working on setting up an appointment for me there. Dr. F said that, obviously, the chemotherapy had not done what we had hoped: to eradicate the cancer. It is highly unlikely that any chemotherapy drug will. We are wasting precious time. Radiation therapy may be an option, but if I do it, any future surgery will be out of the question.

"Let the morning bring me word of your unfailing love, for I have put my trust in you. Show me the way I should go, for to you I lift up my soul." Psalm 143:8

He went on to say that another surgery may be an option. The procedure would essentially mean removing any and all "stuff" that is left in my abdomen area. Details are sketchy to my untrained mind, but I understand enough to know that it would be a huge risk, and even if it is successful, would require a radical life change...definitely not what I want to do.

I went on this afternoon to the infusion room for a round of chemo. While it is not shrinking the cancer, it may be stabilizing it enough to satisfy Dr. F until I can get to MDA. The Human Q-Tip was racing around, and there was a gentleman several cubicles over who completely disregarded the TV volume rule. Everyone on the second floor could hear his Spanish soap opera. I spent most of my time there feeling like an outsider looking in. I was thinking to myself, "Don't these people know that I AM DYING?!? But they are still just acting like everything is normal...tending to patients and watching television and filling prescriptions, and my whole world was just shattered. Again." "Yet I am always with you; you hold me by my right hand. You guide me with your counsel, and afterward you will take me into glory. Whom have I in heaven but you? And earth has nothing

I desire besides you. My flesh and my heart may fail, but God is the strength of my heart and my portion forever." Psalm 73:17

A lot of things changed today. I went to the hospital this morning feeling cautious, but still hopeful. Tonight, hope is hard to find. Time is a precious commodity. If I do nothing—if the option for chemotherapy is taken away and I choose to not go forward with surgery, in a matter of months the cancer can grow in such a way that I will be in an emergency situation that I will not survive. I was surprised today. In all the scenarios I imagined, it never occurred to me that my doctor would say, "I can't do anything else for you. We have exhausted all of our resources" without actually saying it.

> I the Lord do not change. So you, O descendants of Jacob, are not destroyed. (Malachi 3:6)

God wasn't surprised today. He knew. He has known all along. Tonight, while my heart is breaking all over again, He knows what lies ahead. He knows what my choices are. He knows the number of the days of my life and how many breaths I have left to take. I don't feel like rejoicing tonight. I am not lifting my voice in song or raising my hands in worship. What I am doing is telling Him how I feel. How I need more time with my little cowboys. How I hated the tears in my mom's eyes and the look on my husband's face in that doctor's office today. I am shaking my proverbial fist toward the heavens and asking WHY??? But I am also soaking up the Truth. I can find comfort in knowing that while my little world is changing faster than I can keep up with, God is unchanging. Today, yesterday, forever. He promised to remain exactly the same. I believe Him. I don't understand Him, but I believe Him.

> There is surely a future hope for you, and your hope will not be cut off. (Proverbs 23:18)

Bottling It Up

Wednesday, March 13, 2013

Dear Cowboys, It is quiet in our house tonight. I am recovering from what is likely the last chemo treatment I will have, and you are spending your Spring Break week in West Texas with your grandparents. It is nearly too quiet. Your absence makes it easier for me to get in my much-needed nap time, but honestly, I miss the sounds of you slamming doors, rummaging through the pantry (because you are always hungry!), and shouting up and down the stairs. It is lonely here without you. I've been doing a lot of thinking, processing, and praying with the three of you at the forefront of my mind and heart over the last few days. It is exhausting work, being down in the trenches battling it out with God. He and I don't see eye to eye on a few things, but we certainly agree on this: You three little cowboys are wonderfully made and deeply loved. Mema has been great over the last few days to send me some pictures and videos so that I can keep up with what you're doing on your vacation, and I don't feel quite so lonely for you. Indeed, each one makes me smile. You know what I wish? I wish that I could bottle up days like today for you. Days where you chase goats in a brother rodeo and laugh your heads off. Days where you dare each other to try a little polar swimming, Texas style. Days where you are carefree and lighthearted. Days where you are not burdened or hurting. I want to capture THAT in a bottle, label it, and set it up on a shelf somewhere where it will be safe until the time comes that you might need it again.

I'm afraid that there is such a time that is coming, precious loves. I can barely stand the very idea of it. But tonight, in our quiet house, I am asking God to protect your tender hearts for just a while longer. I am begging him for a little more time—a few more days of goat rodeos and playing outside and being little boys. And of course, always, asking and believing for the miracle that will let me be the mom I want to be for you. But you know what the real miracle is? It's that I got to be your mom in the first place. God could have given you to anyone—but he picked me. I am the luckiest lady in the whole world. I love you to the moon and back. Love, Mom

The Monster Within

Saturday, March 23, 2013

THIS WEEK I TRAVELED TO Houston to follow Dr. F's advice: "Get to MD Anderson as quickly as possible." My parents live only about 20 minutes from the MDA campus, which is very convenient. The day before my scheduled appointment, Mom and I were reading through the pile of reports that summarize the last pitiful nine months of my life, when a great idea struck me: I could try to load the accompanying imaging discs (PET and CT scans) on the laptop and maybe I could see with my own eyes what is going on in there. My mom, for the record, thought this was a terrible idea. I was never that great at biology, and I couldn't decipher the CT slices. (Yes, slices. That is not a typo.) But my most recent PET scan…well. That's a different story. It was fascinating in a creepy kind of way. I watched as the screen slowly revealed my brain, my head, my spine, my arms, and my legs. It spun me around in a perfect 360 degree rotation. With a few lucky clicks here and there, I was able to dissect the images until I was staring at IT. Like a terrible Rorschach print, The Sickness—my cancer—seemed to glare at me with the blackest, angriest eyes I have ever seen. In that second, it went from being an obscure thing to almost taking on a personality. He is angry. He is fierce. He is scary. He is tough. I call him Monster. One look was enough. The next day I delivered those discs, along with the written reports, to Dr. B. My curiosity, if that's what you want to call it, is satisfied. The appointment at MDA went as well as it could have, under the circumstances. I learned that without a doubt, Monster is classified as "chemo-resistant." Um, yeah. I have gone through five chemo drugs in five years, and he keeps finding his way back. There will be no more chemotherapy from this point on. That feels good, because chemo is miserable, and it feels scary, because chemo is how you fight cancer. I also learned that Monster should not be treated with radiation or further surgery, at least for the time being. Both are high-risk and present opportunities for new difficulties to arise. Surgery, in particular, would be nothing less than life-altering, and still, there would be no guarantee for a favorable outcome. That doesn't seem to leave many choices, does it? That's what I was thinking. I told you that Monster is tough. Here's the plan: I am returning to MDA next week for further testing. Those ultra-specific scans will tell Dr. B exactly where Monster is in relation to certain things so that she can make a decision about treatment that will (hopefully) not cause further damage to my insides. Make sense? I know. Sigh. There are, according to Dr. B, a few medication options for treatment. One that she is considering attacks the blood vessels of the cancer cells. Another one is a type of hormone therapy. Really, though, there were two main things that Dr. B said to me during our visit that mattered significantly. She said: "How are the boys?" and "Don't give up." Don't give up. That was just seconds after she informed me that Monster's main body part (he has about 4-5) is the size of a baseball. Minutes after I told her that I can, for the first time since 2007, feel the cancer inside my body. I wonder if she could look into my eyes and see how tired I am. I'm sure she could see straight through my brave facade and knew how sick I am of being sick. But maybe, mom to mom, she understood that every breath, no matter how hard it seems, is one more I get to share with my boys. For them, the fight goes on.

Non-Insomniac Blogging

Friday, March 29, 2013

My doctor says that rest is essential for healing. My insomnia, while somewhat useful for blogging purposes, is not helping my case against cancer. She wired an Rx for an increased dose of Ambien over to Walgreens, and POOF! I'm sleeping through the night…well, I'm sleeping better, anyway.

That doesn't keep my brain from observing, thinking, and wanting to state the obvious out loud. So, without further explanation or ado, I present to you the first edition of non-insomniac blogging:

- I have flown to Houston and back twice in the last week. I don't know how regular business travelers do it! I woke up in my own parents' house and barely could remember where I was.
- Waiting for one flight, I entered the terminal and sat down next to a normal looking business man. I glanced over at him and was shocked to see that he was knitting. I think he was making a scarf. When the flight was called, he packed up his creation, his knitting needles, and his

- ball of yarn into a Hudson News bag—and he blended right in with the crowd. Well played, sir. Well played.
- It would be awesome if there were moving sidewalks everywhere we went.
- I always scan the crowd sitting in the terminal to see who I want to sit by. I eliminate anyone who is too talkative, dressed too nice (read: 5-inch heels) or too shabby (read: pajama pants), stressed out business people, women who are loudly arguing with their husbands on their cell phones, and anyone who is angrily watching CSPAN on the terminal television set (although it is on mute). Yikes.
- Although I am not Catholic, I think I am a fan of the new pope. He seems to be very humble and not swayed by the perks of the papacy. I also think he bears a strong resemblance to Paul Shaffer from the CBS Orchestra on Late Night with David Letterman.
- I had this old commercial stuck in my head the other day: You can't watch that without thinking: Two all beef patties, special sauce, lettuce, cheese, pickles, onions, on a sesame seed bun!
- Hamburgers have been few and far between for me since my last surgery. It's a shame.
- In a small waiting room, manners matter.
- The radiology department was running about an hour behind when I was there for testing. That was unfortunate, but at least I had this cuteness sitting across from me: He was playing a game on his cell phone. Bloop…Blooop…Bloooooop. Smile.
- I met a man with breast cancer.
- Nurse: Are you a water drinker?
- Redneck Patient: I'm a beer drinker. Does that count?
- I was surprised to see Smoky Robinson on American Idol. I truly thought he was dead.

- Nine hours after I left Houston, my cousin had her long-awaited baby. Welcome to the world, Evie! I already love you and I can't WAIT to meet you in person.
- I would love to quit my job as a cancer patient and travel with the Mary Poppins tour. Magical.
- My third grade class picture is circulating on Facebook. As if life isn't hard enough.
- Reese the Niece has her first little hairdo:
- Successfully rising to the challenge of entertaining themselves without screen time, there are right now three little boys in our downstairs bathroom telling ghost stories with the lights off. I just heard one of them say, "It's my turn to sit on the toilet!" Ah—boys.

Alive and Well

Monday, April 15, 2013

IT HAS BEEN FIVE WEEKS since my last chemotherapy treatment. It has been three weeks since debate began among several doctors in a few different specialties in a couple of separate hospitals regarding what the status of The Sickness is. The testing has been uncomfortable and inconvenient. The waiting has been nearly unbearable. (Do you know how hard it is to be productive if you are carrying a phone in one hand every waking hour of the day, waiting for it to ring?!?) The professional disagreements have been confusing and worrisome. Finally, FINALLY today the final answer came. Monster is alive and well inside of me. Scans are just pictures, and pictures can be tricky. But biopsies do not lie. I wasn't really surprised that the biopsy was positive. What surprised me today was the emotion I felt. I've been in this fight long enough now that I thought I had developed nerves of steel. Great sadness washed over me as I listened to Nurse Allyson deliver the news. I realized that I had allowed myself to imagine a cancer-free me, and my sadness was the equivalent of disappointment. I believe in miracles. I believe that the same God who raised Lazarus from the dead, turned the water into wine, and made the blind man see can also make me whole and well. I believe that He is good. I do not understand why He does not allow that healing to take place. I do not understand. And oh, how I desperately want to understand it. I would give almost anything just for the assurance that all of this suffering—mine and my family's—is not in vain. But I suppose that would not really be faith, would it? Blessed assurance, Jesus is mine.

Facing the Future

Sunday, April 21, 2013

THIS UPDATE IS A HARD one to write. I've been dreading it and have, in fact, been putting it off. However, procrastination is not going to change the facts, so it's time to put them out there for you, my friends, to know. Monster lives. He resists chemotherapy. He has come back to life after four major surgeries designed to destroy him. He is too big for radiation. He is too aggressive and unpredictable for other common treatments. He is a threat to other body parts and functions, which, once damaged, can not be reversed and could be life-threatening. His location within my body makes nontraditional treatments questionable at best, and more like out of the question. Monster is not going away. In the last few weeks, I've had to make a difficult decision. Since the debate was settled with a positive biopsy result, it has become clear that Monster intends to stay. I have to change my thinking, my prayers, my outlook, my plans…my LIFE!…to accommodate that. After much consideration, prayer, counsel, and discussion, I have decided to opt out of further chemotherapy treatments. While chemo may be maintaining Monster to some degree, it is not shrinking him and certainly not getting rid of him! What it is doing is stealing from me. It is stealing 3–4 perfectly good days every week when I can not function like ME. It is stealing my energy. It is stealing my spirit, my joy, and most of all, it is stealing precious time. If the rest of my time on this earth is going to be shared with Monster—and right now, it appears that it will be—then I must make that time quality. I want to spend that time being ME. I am not a cancer patient. I am a wife and a mom. I am a daughter and a sister. I am a granddaughter and an auntie. I am a friend. I am a follower of Jesus Christ. I love music. I like to laugh, good food, Mary Poppins, animals, wise sayings, mystery books, Target, and flip flops. I must have my morning cup of coffee, my toenails painted, and a little bit of alone time every day. These are the things that make my world turn. I might have cancer, but it does not have me. I have started on a new medication that I can take at home, once a day. It blocks estrogen production, thereby starving the cancer cells. (Monster eats estrogen.) This pill is similar to the med that I took from 2010–2012, when Monster was on vacation. The hope is that he will go on vacation again…this time for a long, long time. Let's be clear: This is not me giving up. This is not me throwing in the towel or denying the possibility of God granting an 11th hour miracle. This is me, facing the very real idea that I may not see my babies grow their first mustaches, go on their first dates, or nurse their first broken hearts. I may not live long enough to be at my sons' high school graduation ceremonies. I may not be here to dance at their weddings or rock my grand babies. I need to be prepared for anything, so I want to get busy LIVING! "She is clothed with strength and dignity, and she laughs without fear of the future." Proverbs 31:25 Please, Lord, let it be said of me. P.S. I don't know how much dignity a lady with a bird on her head can possibly muster, but it was a beautiful afternoon to go to the zoo with my 3 favorite boys!

High and Stormy Gale

Tuesday, June 25, 2013

EARLY THIS MORNING WE DROPPED the cowboys off with a friend so they could go to VBS and we nervously fought rush hour traffic to get to Dr. F's office. We had every reason to be anxious. I had a CT scan on Friday. The scan shows at least four new tumors that have developed since April. The existing masses are enlarged, and there is some growth into lymph nodes. Four new tumors. Three little cowboys.

When darkness veils His lovely face I rest on His unchanging grace. There are two choices:

1. Surgery.

    Further examination led Dr. F to solemnly tell us that surgery would be difficult. The tumors are growing at such a rapid rate that they are jam-packed in my body. He believes that there are parts that are even attached to bone. Surgery would require a 2-week hospital stay, followed by a lengthy recovery at home. The result would mean a huge lifestyle change for me, and there is no guarantee that such an operation would be successful in eradicating Monster.

2. Nothing.

I can continue as I am, treating the pain and other symptoms as they come along with medication.

In every high and stormy gale my anchor holds within the veil. Neither seems like a good option to me. I don't even have a backup plan anymore, as my team at M.D. Anderson has done everything they can do for me. Dr. F suggested that I might consider making a trip to New York to Memorial Sloan Kettering Hospital, to seek any resources that might not be at our disposal here in Texas. Part of me thinks that is a great idea! Part of me thinks that if I didn't get it at MDA, I won't get it at MSK. And a third, hidden, terrible part of me wants to stick out her tongue and stamp her foot at the very idea that her first trip to New York City would be on Monster's behalf! Really...the nerve!!! His oath, His covenant, His blood, support me in the whelming flood. This isn't just a little summer shower of "oh, drat." This is a full-fledged, gale-force, torrential deluge of "DAMN IT!!!" This is a monstrosity of a storm. These are rising flood waters that threaten everything I hold dear. This squall refuses to be quieted or calmed. This is my life. When all around my soul gives way He then is all my hope and stay. All around me today everything fell apart...again. I went into that little room not even expecting a miracle. I had only hoped that Monster might have just been contained for the last few months. To find out that he is growing faster than Little Middle (who is eating us out of house and home, by the way) was like taking a sucker punch to the gut. But God. ...So loved Allyson that He gave His only son. So that no matter what I come across in this broken old world: heartache, loss, sickness, fear—I have hope. On Christ the Solid Rock I stand, all other ground is sinking sand, All other ground is sinking sand.

Making Decisions

Monday, July 08, 2013

THERE HAS BEEN A LOT of talking, praying, and weighing of options going on around here. Hubby took a few days off work last week, and we spent much of that time discussing our future. We have made some decisions. I will not have another debulking surgery. The possible benefits are minuscule when compared to the probable risks. I want to spend my time not suffering in bed, but making memories with my family. With Dr. F's blessing, I have scheduled two appointments. I hesitate to use the word "final," but it certainly feels like they are final appointments. Last chances. End-of-the-road. The first one I went to today at UT Southwestern here in Dallas. I saw a doctor whose career specialty is advanced gyn cancers. She was extremely generous with her time and I could see compassion in her eyes. She wanted to give me good news. There was talk of pathology review and tumor classification, but in the end, she confirmed what we already know. My Monster is rare—less than 10% of all ovarian cancer patients experience this sort of evolution of cancer. It is strong, mean, and without a miracle, it will be nearly impossible to eradicate. The second appointment I made will take place at

Memorial Sloane-Kettering Cancer Center in New York on July 22. My medical records were forwarded to MSK, and after review, my request for an appointment was approved. There is much to be done in preparation for that appointment: paperwork must be gathered, pathology slides from all four of my previous surgeries must be overnighted to the clinic, and arrangements must be made. I have not anticipated earth-shattering revelations from either of these doctors. Quite the opposite, actually. After years of disappointing—no, crushing—tests, reports, and appointments, I know better than to have high expectations. Instead, my ambition is simple: I want to be settled. I want to know without a doubt that I have done everything reasonable to fight a good fight. I want to be able to look my husband, my little cowboys, and my parents in the eye and be confident that I did my best for them. Make no mistake, friends. This is not resignation, nor am I giving up. I believe that God still does miracles all the time, and that He can heal. We continue to pray for that miracle. And I also believe that God has a good plan for me—even if it is cancer. These are scary days, yet I feel peace. That is a good gift from a good God.

> "Faith is deliberate confidence in the character of God whose ways you may not understand at the time."
>
> —Oswald Chambers

A Different Kind of Trial

Thursday, July 25, 2013

A LIFELONG DREAM CAME TRUE this week when I landed in New York's La Guardia Airport. I've always wanted to go see the sights, watch the people, taste the food, even sniff the smells for myself.

Of course, I have always thought that I would travel to NYC for fun. My reason for this particular trip was about as far from fun as I could get. In fact, I went to New York this week for a doctor appointment. A last-ditch, end-of-the-road, please-God-let-this-be-the-one doctor appointment. The third oncology specialist in a month. I am sick to death of doctors offices. I am fed up with waiting rooms. I never want to hold another clipboard, record my surgical history, report my allergy to morphine, or provide my insurance card again. Ever. I despise thin white sheets, because they are NOT soft, warm, or sufficient coverings. Nonetheless I found myself on Monday morning in a wing of Memorial Sloan-Kettering Cancer Center, not far from Times Square, anxiously holding a clipboard on my lap and coaxing my insurance card from its safe place in my wallet. I checked my phone one more time to get a glimpse of the sweet faces of my three little cowboys. It reminded me of how far I had come. Instead of bolting for the anonymity of the city streets, I stayed put and allowed myself to be led to an exam room. My parents and my Seester had accompanied me, and their presence calmed me. The doctor was timely, and got right down to business. She had reviewed all of my records (and believe me, there was plenty to review). She repeated much of what we had already heard: The Monster is evil. It is aggressive. It is really hanging in there! Surgery is risky and not recommended at this point. Then she said something different: "We have a new clinical trial that I think you would be eligible for." *Disclaimer: Scientists are a different breed. I am not a scientist. What Dr. G tried to explain in our time together seriously made my head swirl. She made me think of my statistics professor in college, when all I wanted to do was pass the class—not even make a good grade, just pass—because listening to him talk was like trying to comprehend a second language. I am a mother. I understand snot and blood and poop and dirt. I do not understand cancer. Read on at your own risk.* The clinical trial is a phase 3 trial, meaning that it is in the final phase of research before it can be presented for approval to the FDA. The goal of a phase 3 clinical trial is to see if an investigational drug works better (or has fewer side effects) than the standard treatment. This particular drug, known as MEK162, is an inhibitor. Instead of killing actual cancer cells, it targets the cell growth pathway that is specific to low-grade serous ovarian cancer. MEK162 is an oral medication that is taken twice a day. Likely side effects include skin irritations, stomach issues, fatigue, fluid retention, and increases in muscle enzymes. There are other side effects, but they are farther down on the "likely to happen" scale. Now for the tricky part. This clinical trial is randomized. As is true with all scientific experiments, there must be a control group. All trial participants will be randomized by a computer system to receive either the MEK162 medication OR one of the standard first-line chemotherapies. 2/3 of participants will receive the MEK inhibitor; 1/3 will receive chemo. What does that mean for me? Well, I've already done all of the chemotherapies that are on the list. All with no success. I'm not too eager to go back and do them again. Actually, if I got it in my head to try chemo again, I would just call up dear old Dr. F and say so. He would make it happen. It's absurd, and I digress. I have absolutely nothing to lose by taking part in this clinical trial. I am already facing the worst case scenario. What can a little phase 3 pill hurt? I have already made the phone call to the site here in DFW that will administer the trial. These things are never simple, of course, and I anticipate frustrating days ahead with more clipboards and more paper-thin white sheets. God has been good, though, to answer my prayer for clear direction and to grant me peace in the middle of my life's biggest storm. I am thankful for this sliver of hope. I am thankful that I serve a big God. And I am thankful for the wide open spaces and the drive friendly laws in TEXAS!

Mad

Thursday, August 01, 2013

DEAR CANCER, AS YOU KNOW, I am not much of an activist. I don't raise funds or go to health expos. I only attend one 5k walk each year (although I walk with defiant pride!). I have other ways of expressing my feelings. Today, I am really mad at you! You are a sneaky, meaner-than-mean SOB. You have no boundaries for your prey: rich, poor, old, young, male, or female. So I guess I shouldn't have been so surprised when I received the unwelcome news of my longtime friend's breast cancer diagnosis this afternoon. I am not usually at a loss for words, but this message left me speechless. But not for long. No, sir. I picked up my phone and I dialed across the miles. The second I heard her voice, it came back to me: how I felt six years ago. How I was her when a doctor said to me, "I have bad news. It's cancer." How you changed my life. And you know what? I liked my life. I didn't invite you. I didn't want you. I DO NOT LIKE YOU. Yet, you refuse to leave me alone. What's the deal? What is it about me that you think is so great? Is it my affinity for musicals and carbohydrates? My nifty sense of humor? My ability to make up songs on the spot? And my sweet friend. I know why I love her, but what could you possibly want with her? Is it her Job-like patience? Her fun-loving spirit of adventure? Her affection for snow cones?!? With one phone call, she was pinned with the unwanted pink ribbon. Blah. Pink, teal, whatever the color...it isn't a badge of honor. It's not a privilege to fight this fight. I, and now my dear friend, and millions just like us, fight because we have to. Because you invade our bodies, but even more than that: you attack our lives. You interfere with every. single. aspect of everything until there are more questions than there are answers. Not only am I mad at you for invading, but I am FURIOUS at you for the questions. Today my counselor (and I would like to insert that my need for a counselor is also your fault) gently and graciously guided me through nearly an hour of gut-wrenching talk of ...have I done enough? when is enough enough? how much is too much? how will they know how much I love them? will they remember? does he understand that he is our everything? should I be scared? can I be peaceful?...and so on and so on. The tears flowed fast and furious. The counselor knows that I am mad at you and she says that's OK. So there. You suck. This world is broken, yes, and sin-filled, and I still don't think that is a good enough reason for you to be here. Be gone! Get out! Maybe I'll become a cancer activist after all and take up the cause. You've done enough damage, both inside and out. I'm sick of you. Fed up, Allyson Confidential to M: So, today was a bad day. And there will be some more bad days. But hear me loud and clear, sister: you are not alone!!! There is no way that I am going to sit over here and let you walk down this road unassisted. I KNEW all this cancer stuff would come in handy someday! :) It's okay to be scared, and it's okay to be mad (obviously!), as long as you remember the three things:

1) God loves us. 2) God is always in control. 3) God is good. You are the daughter of a big, big God who is holding you in the palm of his big, big hand. And you have a slightly crazy friend who will do just about anything for you. Anytime, day or night. Any reason. You are loved. Oh yeah—-let's hit up Bahama Buck's, okay? My treat.

Rain On

Friday, August 09, 2013

THERE IS THUNDER RUMBLING OUTSIDE and the sky is turning dark. There is a storm brewing out there, and that is just fine with me. A Friday night thunderstorm is the perfect way to end this week. Our dryer broke. All the little lights come on, but when I push the start button, the dumb thing goes "beep beep." Every. Single. Time. "Beep beep." "Beep beep." "BEEP BEEP." My techno-nerd hubby used the Google and got some ideas. He ordered a new part, which was delivered today. So far, no luck. "Beep beep." In the meantime…it's no secret that I detest laundry even when all the machines are working. You can only imagine the joy it has been to drape each individual sock, towel, and little-boy undie over the shower, tub, trampoline, swing, fireplace, and finally, my friend Krystal's drying rack. If you see us out and about and we look a little wrinkled and/or crusty, you'll know why. The location for the clinical trial has been narrowed down for me because nothing else is available. Looks like I will be traveling to Oklahoma, where the wind comes sweeping down the plain! The first step is to meet with the trial doctor to discuss my history and make a final decision about my eligibility to participate. That meeting will take place on Monday. Although I fully realize that this clinical trial has the potential to be the hope that I have asked God for, I am having a hard time being cheerful about it. For one thing, I will endure a rigorous screening process made up of multiple tests that for some reason can not be all done in one trip to Oklahoma City. I do not understand this. For another thing, it is possible that I will go through the screening and randomization processes, only to be informed that I can not take the trial drug. "But here," they will say. "We would like to offer you some lovely Taxol as a consolation prize. 100% guaranteed to make your hair fall out! Tried and failed to cure cancer! Congratulations!" That would be neat-o. By the way, in case that scenario should occur (and there is a 1 in 3 chance that it will), this is what I will do: WALK AWAY. I am not doing chemotherapy again. 5 drugs in 3 years. I guess you can safely say that I am not chemo-compatible. Here is another reason that I hate this week. This conversation happened: Little Middle: What time will Mr. Dad be home? Me: Around 5:30. Little Middle: Can I call him and see what time he will get here? Me: No! I just told you when he'll be here! Little Middle: (making pouting face and crossing arms across chest) Me: You sure are anxious for Daddy to get home. (Teasing) Why does he get to be the fun parent? Little Middle: (Serious face) Because you're always sick. Ugh. He said it the honest, this-is-what-I-really-think way that kids say stuff. He wasn't trying to be hurtful. Just real. Then today, we had another big blow—one I'm not quite ready to write about, but you can believe me when I tell you that I deserved that glass of wine I drank at almost-5:00. AND my darling cowboys ran off to their friends' house with my laptop and all of the leftover Chick-Fil-A ketchup and Buffalo sauce packets in their backpack. You know, for the monster movie they were making. Special effects...very, very special. I hope it rains. I hope the heavens open wide and it pours down. I hope there is thunder and lightning to match my mood. I love a rainy night...but not a stormy life.

"If She Liked Me Any More, She'd Sic the Dogs on Me."

Friday, September 13, 2013

OVER THE RED RIVER AND just across the state line, things are quiet. Too quiet. It has been nearly five weeks since I signed consent to participate in the MEK162 clinical trial. On that day, the researchers seemed thrilled to have me. The head doctor was extremely interested in Monster and our history together. She promised that they would work quickly to obtain and dissect a tissue block from one of my debulking surgeries. That did indeed happen, but with unfortunate results: There were not enough cancer cells in the sample to qualify as measurable. Monster did not meet their strict criteria.

I was slightly confused, but of course I granted my permission for them to try again. A second block of tissue was FedExed to Oklahoma, and the investigational researchers got busy doing their thing. After another week of waiting, I called and was given news that I did not care to hear. Sample #2 was also a bust—the necessary slides were easily made, but none of them contained enough tumor.

"How can that be?" I asked Michelle the research nurse. "There is plenty of tumor in there! I can feel it!"

Michelle suspects that during each of the surgeries, the doctor cut out the tumors (which he was supposed to), but did such a good job that there was very little left over for remaining tissue. In other words, I was greatly debulked. That is good for surgery, but bad for research.

I should have started treatment by now. I need to have started treatment by now. Monster has made his presence known in a few new and frightening ways in my body. Dr. F says that there is nothing to be done but to proceed with treatment as quickly as possible. After all this waiting and receiving discouraging news, I was not quite prepared to make the decision that was presented to me yesterday. I could a) be released back to Dr. F to receive the standard of care (read: chemotherapy), or b) travel to Oklahoma for a scan and intense biopsy. I have already taken every chemo drug that is considered "standard of care" for ovca patients. Each drug was unsuccessful. I chose to pack my suitcase and go north.

Of course, nothing can be simple or easy. The appointments must be done at certain times of the day with certain medical personnel. That means more waiting for me while Oklahoma tries to get their act together. With any luck, I will be able to travel next week. Through all of this, Monster lives. He is such a pain (literally!). I think of him as being like those animated germs in the Mucinex commercials. You know, the ones where they set up homes inside the sick person's body? They stay there, relaxing in their easy chairs and inviting their friends in, until the miracle Mucinex comes in and kicks them back to the curb. I feel like Monster has claimed my body as his own personal space. He doesn't care that he is creating chaos. He only cares that he has found a good spot, and he is fighting to stay put.

Although I am frustrated and discouraged, I continue to fight. I get out of bed each morning, determined not to let Monster change my life, or even cramp my style. I have three very good reasons, after all, to fight back...they call me Mom.

Oklahoma (Not) Okay

Saturday, September 28, 2013

I HAVE JUST RETURNED FROM a whirlwind 27-hour road trip to Oklahoma City. I am sitting in my quiet-for-now house, absorbing the familiar surroundings and a little bit wishing I had never left in the first place.

I left Texas, my Texas yesterday morning with my mom. Can I just take a minute and tell you how great my mom is? She holds down a full-time job in which she pours herself into other people. But…she is Mom and Nana first. We all know it. She insists on attending each doctor visit, regardless of time, location, or convenience. She has traveled literally across the country with me on the search for a cure, and she is my #1 cheerleader. She has lived in my home, taken care of my family, and stepped in for me when I simply could not do for myself. She created an Allyson playlist just for this trip with my favorite tunes, and we listened to it going and coming. There is no one who gives more, expects less, or has a bigger heart. I love you, Mom.

Back to the story…Mom and I drove the 3 hours to OKC and made it there with a little time to spare. We checked in to our hotel and I managed to get in a quick nap before we were in the car again headed for the OU Medical district. I have to say this for Oklahoma: The CT scan I did there was the easiest, most pleasant (if such a thing can be pleasant) radiology experience that I have had. The staff was efficient and kind, AND, instead of the terrible barium drink, they only asked me to drink a regular bottle of water before the test. It made for a much, much more comfortable exam. I was in and out of there in record time. I didn't leave empty-handed, either! The sweet nurse loaded me down with a fresh bottle of water, a granola bar (to make up for not eating for 6+ hours), and a thank you card. Texas, take note! There IS a better way!

We had been back in our hotel room for just a few minutes when my phone rang. It was the research nurse calling with results. The scan had disqualified me from the clinical trial. Just like that, I'm out. Yes, there is cancer in there. But instead of being one (or more) large masses, there is what is known as "papillary smattering." It means that there are lots of small pieces of cancer just…everywhere. Monster is having a block party.

I couldn't help it. I cried. I have found that the longer the fight wears on, the less I tend to cry. I suppose I'm used to it. But never before have I wanted for the cancer to show up bigger or plainer on a scan…and the one time I need it to, it does THIS?!? The news was more than my heart could bear.

We spent a long and noisy night in OK, thanks to a rambunctious group of retirees who stopped in during their bus tour (Tour of what? I am still wondering.) and the truck stop next door to our hotel. Neither of us was sad to pack up and check out. On our way out of town, we stopped back in at the medical building so I could retrieve the CT disc and copies of the report. The research nurse met me in the lobby and provided this tidbit of encouragement: There will be a site for the MEK162 study opening in several months closer to my home. By that time, perhaps my cancer will have grown to meet the criteria size.

Yes, and perhaps the farmer and the cowman should be friends.

Three Little Cowboys

I did not cry when I finally saw the Red River in the rearview mirror. I would sum up my visit to Oklahoma by borrowing the words of a friend I once traveled with: "This state is a complete disaster." (**No offense, of course, to my friends with OK ties. You can still feel free to eat your fried pies, cheer for your football team, and house your law firms inside your churches.)

So what now? Good question. Before I even left Oklahoma, I called Dr. F's office. He again offered to set up chemotherapy, just to give me something to try. I again declined, noting that if I have any more chemo—no matter where or what—I will have zero chance of EVER getting into the MEK162 trial, as I have already maxed out what they allow in that area. Not to mention that any chemotherapy that is available to me as a "standard of care" I have already taken and found no success. He was not surprised. Dr. F suggested that I might try calling MD Anderson again, essentially starting over there with another doctor. MDA has clinical trials that are exclusive to their organization. For that reason, I will take his advice.

When Goliath was little, he loved to play hide-and-seek. I would hide, usually with a baby brother on my hip and Abby Dog following closely, and he would look for me. Some days I would deviate from the usual hiding places—in the shower, behind the laundry room door, underneath a blanket in the closet—and he would have to work harder to find me. If it was taking too long to find me, he would just stop looking. At age 3, he didn't have the courtesy to call out and let me know he was done…he just quit. It was too hard, it was taking too long, he couldn't find what he was looking for. (Would have been nice to know on that day I hid in the dirty laundry hamper. I couldn't stand up straight for two days!)

I feel like that little Goliath now. I am so frustrated! The search has gone on for a really long time. I just want to wave the white flag of surrender and be done. I want to get back to what I want to do and forget what I have to do.

Allyson Hendrickson

This week's disappointment has brought back the old question that has nagged for such a long while: What does God want? I rarely do the "why me?" thing; I tend to think instead "why NOT me?" I know that there is nothing about me that is better or more deserving than anyone else. But why the ongoing suffering? "Suffering" is a heavy word, but there is not a better one to describe the physical pain I have, but also the emotional anguish that I carry—and others share. Sometimes I think that this would be so different if I had never married the man I love… or if we had not had children…or if my "Original Five" weren't so close…or if… I were alone. I HATE knowing that I am causing pain for others. If I could walk away…

I would get exactly nowhere. Cancer would still be there, suffering would follow me. It is hard to follow God when you don't understand Him, isn't it? It's hard to know what to do when you feel forgotten. It is hard to trust when you feel let down.

"He has shown you, O man, what is good. And what does the Lord require of you? To act justly, to love mercy, and to walk humbly with your God." Micah 6:8

Lord, help me to do what is good. I want to walk with you, and I need your strength in these difficult days. I don't understand cancer, I don't like it, and I would love it if you would erase it completely from my body. But I know that you have a plan for me and I believe that it is good. Please help me to trust you. Show me where to go and what to do next, and then lead the way!… because I will follow you wherever you go. Amen.

C Is for Cancer

Tuesday, October 08, 2013

It cracks me up when I go to a medical office and I have to do the assessment with the nurse. They're all basically the same: current complaint, history, vitals, and then she will ask, "Do you have any other conditions that we should be aware of?" My answer: "Nope. Aside from the pesky cancer, I am perfectly healthy."

It's an answer that came in handy on Sunday morning when I found myself in the emergency room. I started feeling more cancer-y (yes, I just created a new adjective) than usual late last week. Friday afternoon was a rapid decline of stomach-related symptoms and pain that refused to be controlled with meds, even heavy duty prescriptions. I had more of the same on Saturday, growing progressively weaker and dehydrated. By 8 a.m. on Sunday I knew that I had to get help. We called ahead to Dr. F's office and Hubby drove me to the ER. I have only been in the ER once before, on the day that Monster moved in and set up shop. That was six years ago. It hasn't changed much. Even though we had called my doctor ahead of time, I am an established patient at the hospital, AND I was miserable, it took more than two hours to get past triage, and I didn't see an actual doctor until I had been there for seven hours. In spite of feeling terrible, though, the wait gave me plenty of time for people watching. One quartet was particularly interesting. The gentleman who turned out to be the patient (it took me a while to figure that out!) was dressed in a heavy camouflage hunting coat. Now, we had a cold front come through DFW, but this coat was crazy. It was the I-am-going-out-in-a-snowstorm-to-kill-a-wild-animal coat, not a there's-finally-a-chill-in-the-air jacket. Coat Man was accompanied by an entourage of characters who appeared to be family members... maybe his mother and siblings? Mama was probably so distressed about her sick son that she rushed out without her bra. It was frighteningly absent beneath her straight-from-the-junior-section Tinkerbell t-shirt. Coat Man's brother might have been equally distracted, because he forgot to pull his pants all the way up. He also never removed his sunglasses. For hours. Coat Man's sister won the prize, though, because she forgot to get dressed AT ALL. She seemingly fell out of bed and straight into the car that brought her brother to the hospital. Had I been brave enough, I might have given her this nugget of advice: You might receive better service in this fine health care establishment if you wear undergarments with your paper-thin white t-shirt, don pants that are NOT decorated with flannel Cookie Monsters, and leave your bathrobe with holes in the elbows at home. Oh, and please just try to last longer than 5 minutes before you go outside for another smoke. Good grief.

I finally got called back into a tiny room. I had x-rays done, blood taken, and got fluids going. The sweet nurse gave me injections of pain and anti-nausea meds. After the second round, I felt relief. FINALLY. Turns out that I have a couple of nasty infections. Monster welcomed the visiting germs...he probably offered them lemonade and asked them to stay a while. I walked out of the ER with hefty meds to add to my collection and directions to call my doctor during regular business hours if I needed anything else.

Two days later, I am still feeling blah (but better than Sunday!). Monster and his buddies seem to have their seat belts fastened in their easy chairs in there. Lemonade, anyone? As is my practice, I have been trying to find the proverbial silver lining. First, it was a weekend. As much as I hate it, Hubby was able to step up for full-time Cowboy Duty so I could rest. Second, there is nothing like a crisis to bring the best out in the best people. I've said it so many times, and I will say it again: We have been blessed with some amazing people. They continually stand with us, behind us, and around us—encircling my guys and me with incredible love. This is the body of Christ as it should be…Jesus with skin on.

Finally, and I know this sounds strange, but this weekend was useful as a practice run. Dr. F expects that Monster will culminate his stay by causing obstruction of some vital organs/functions. When that happens—and it is WHEN, not IF—it will be a true, life-threatening emergency. We have a plan of action ready for that occurrence, which begins with me getting to the MCD ER as quickly as possible. Now we know a little more of what to expect, and that is not a bad thing.

C is for cancer. C is also for Cookie Monster and coat and crazy and cry…and cowboys. I despise this disease that I sometimes say is ruining my life. But there are times when I think of all the things I have seen and done and learned because of cancer that I would never have encountered otherwise. And I have just enough sense in my little head to be thankful.

P.S. Highlight of the long, sick weekend: Lengthy FaceTime with Reese the Niece. She showed me her puppy dogs, she took me outside, and she read me her favorite books. The Princess was astonished that Auntie knew 5 Little Monkeys and could do the hand motions with her. Our favorite part, of course, was when "one fell off and bumped his head!" She'd bump her head, I'd bump my head, and then we would laugh at each other. I am so totally in love with that little girl!

Something

Thursday, November 07, 2013

On Monday afternoon, it was raining in Big D. A promised cold front had pushed through (finally!) and brought with it a brisk wind and much-needed rain. It was the perfect afternoon to snuggle up with a warm cup of coffee—pumpkin spice creamer included—and watch the Disney Channel with the cowboys. Ahhhhh. Except…that's not what I was doing on Monday afternoon. I was speeding across Dallas in the cold rain, trying to beat the rush-hour buildup. My hair was a frizzy mess, my makeup was smudged, and my sweater was hanging halfway off because I couldn't decide if I was hot or cold. I was a hot mess, on my way to the airport to catch a plane to Houston.

After weeks of trying, I was finally able to score an appointment at MD Anderson. My regular MDA doctor rejected my request to see her, by flat out telling me that she had nothing to offer. Instead, I was referred over to the Center for Targeted Therapy. The doctor there, Dr. W, was one of those people who makes you feel dumb just by being in the same room with you. Not because she was arrogant or talked down to me; she was just SO SMART! It was almost like she was speaking another language, which I had to struggle to follow. Dr. W also had two assistants: Rosa and Roosevelt. I think that Roosevelt is an awesome name. (Hey, Brother and his Other! Take note! Just in case you want to change your mind…)

So, the culmination of my meeting with Dr. W, Rosa, and Roosevelt resulted in an agreement to do two different things:

1) Molecular mapping. Samples of my tissue will be analyzed at the molecular level. Through this analysis, they should be able to determine the exact abnormalities/defects that cause cells in my body to be "bad" cancerous cells. With that information, they may be able to match me to a specific drug that would not normally fall within my standard of care. For instance, I might have the same abnormalities as another group of patients with liver cancer. I would then be able to be treated with medications for liver cancer. Weird, but interesting.

2) Clinical trial. The molecular profiling will take a while—at least a few months. The trial in question is an "in the meantime" solution—completely different from the Oklahoma fiasco trial. This clinical trial involves 2 drugs, both of which have already been approved by the FDA. One drug has been used for a long time with diabetes patients, the other has been used to treat breast cancer. The trial is testing their efficacy when they are given in combination. Both drugs are given orally.

Now, a few things you should know about this clinical trial: The temptation to dance a jig is pretty huge. Just the fact that she did not dismiss me but instead had some ideas is a cause for celebration! But I need to step back and gather my thoughts before I jump off the cliff of crazy. The truth is that these medications, even if successful, are not designed to be a cure. They are meant to, at best, slow the growth of those wretched bad cells, thereby buying me some more time until, hopefully, there IS a cure. (Worst case scenario, I'll endure funky side effects, but maybe I won't get diabetes or breast cancer.) Knowing that truth reminds me of the sobering fact that cancer is what I have. Unless God changes his mind or intervenes, I will have cancer until I die. It may not always be as big, or as painful, but modern medicine tells me that this is my lot in life. Many have prayed for my healing. And it may still be done, but it has become pretty clear to my medical team (and to myself) that this Monster intends to stay.

I am not publicly declaring my "I am thankful" list this month, but I do have one. While the rest of the world is using social media to advertise what they are thankful for, I am keeping mine private. But on Tuesday afternoon, when my plane landed safely on the runway in Dallas, and I knew I would soon be home with my babies, there was no question about it. I am thankful for something. Something to do. Something to take. Something to aid in my fight. Something instead of nothing.

I don't claim to know God's plan. I don't understand why he chooses to withhold physical healing. I don't like my situation, and there are a lot of days when I don't say, "Your will, not mine." And still...He loves me with a depth that I can not comprehend. He values me to a point that I can not understand. He is faithful to provide for me—whether that be the miraculous healing, or a small "something," He is good.

P.S. This is for sale in the Dallas airport, as if the world needed reminding. Poor taste, Dallas. Seriously.

Monster Madness

Wednesday, November 27, 2013

I HAVE BEEN SITTING ON the counter in my mom's kitchen for the last little bit, popping cherry tomatoes into my mouth like they are the last morsels of food on the planet. That's because I ate next to nothing today. I couldn't eat anything because I was too busy being treated like a cancerous piece of crap. Wanna hear about it? I'm here in Houston, where it is actually cold, ya'll. Well, cold by Houston standards, anyway. I'm wearing a sweater.

It's unheard of. I'm here because I had a crazy lineup of cancer appointments at MD Anderson. I was there from 7:30 a.m. to 4:30 p.m. yesterday, and 9:30 a.m. to 4:30 p.m. today. It's been a long, grueling, unbelievable 48 hours. Yesterday was Test Day. I had blood work done. I did an echocardiogram, an EKG, x-rays, and last but not least, my favorite: The CT Scan. It went ok up until the end when the nurse was trying to start an IV for the CT contrast. She was not able to find a usable vein. She called a friend nurse, who found one, stuck a needle in me, and then watched the vein collapse. Nurse #3 came along, stuck me, failed, and stuck me again. Ow ow ow ow ow ow ouch!!!! After that, they gave up and sent me to the Infusion Therapy department, where I waited an HOUR for a member of "The IV Team" to save the day. Ridiculous. But Super-Craig easily placed the needle and got good blood flow. Once that was done, the test itself was far from enjoyable, but was manageable. This morning I put on my sweater and my tall black boots, and braced myself for the day. Mom and I got to MDA 40 minutes before my first scheduled appointment. I can't go into all the details here—you wouldn't believe it if I did—but it will suffice to tell you that I FINALLY saw a nurse practitioner at 2:30…more than 4 hours after my 10:10 appointment time. Unbelievable. I'm usually a pretty nice lady, but I wasn't feeling all that benevolent this afternoon. So much so, in fact, that I rounded out my day by filing a complaint in the Patient Advocacy department. MDA needs to get it together. The complaint came as a result of someone failing to do their job. We have been waiting for our insurance company to approve the clinical trial. Staff that I spoke with assured me that it would be taken care of by the time my appointment rolled around today. However, when I arrived at MDA today, insurance had approved only one of the two pills that make up the clinical trial. One without the other is useless. (Confidential to all you haters: This is not a political thing, an Obamacare thing, a Democrat thing, or whatever else you want to blame it on. It's just a stupid money thing.) An appeal has been filed, but if Aetna doesn't come to their senses, then the clinical trial is out. I also discovered that under clinical trial rules, if insurance doesn't come through and pay, then all of the tests that I did yesterday will be for nothing. They are only good for a short period of time. After that time is up, I will have to go back and redo every blood draw, heart check, and The Scan. Grrrr. One of the appointments that I had today was with a radiologic oncologist. (Try saying that three times fast!) Interestingly, this is the first appointment I've had with a radiologic onc. Ever. It has never been a viable treatment option—until now. The radiation intern showed unmatched kindness as he explained how it works, and more importantly, why I need it. Monster is growing…really, really fast and really, really big. Dr. Brown displayed the images from yesterday's CT scan. He patiently explained what I was looking at on each frame. What I saw was astonishing, and then was confirmed by the paper report from the radiologist. That report tells of "a large pelvic mass," measuring nearly 10 centimeters at its widest point. The mass, aka "Monster," is tangled up, wrapped around, and filling up every nook and cranny in my lower abdomen. He is even touching my tailbone! Additionally, there are two Monster babies in my lungs—one on the right, and one on the left. With such exponential increases in growth, radiation would be a palliative care option for me. There is some hope that it might help to control the symptoms that Monster has brought along. The always-amazing Nurse Allyson gave me a name of a doctor who works with Dr. F. I'm banking on him agreeing to do the radiation so I can be close to home. Two days before Thanksgiving, and this bombshell was dropped in my lap. It's not a surprise, per se, but there's something about sticking a number on it… 10 centimeters is a big enough space to birth a baby. 10 centimeters is approximately the diameter of a bagel. 10 centimeters roughly measures an average-size man's palm (crosswise). 10 centimeters is the diameter of a wiffle ball. Those are sobering measurements. While I was lying on the table listening to the machine instruct me on when to breathe, I closed my eyes tight. I did not really care to see the fake ceiling tiles that I suppose are meant to be calming. They had lovely cherry blossoms on them.

In my mind, cherry blossoms don't belong in the fifth circle of hell. I chose instead to keep my eyes closed and concentrate on Truth. Snippets of Scripture played through my mind like an old recording: "You are precious in my sight…I will not leave you or forsake you…wherever you go, I am there…when you go through the fire, the flames will not touch you…I know the plans I have for you…I will strengthen you and help you…My yoke is easy and my burden is light…I will lift my eyes to the hills from whence comes my help." Those same pieces of Truth ran through my head as I looked at the pictures of Monster. His ugliness, his scariness stared back at me through the screen and made my heart beat faster. Even the doctor said, "He is angry." But I know this: Whether Monster is the size of a bagel or a beach ball, my God is bigger. My God is stronger. My God will not leave me to do this by myself. Every day brings me a little bit closer to the reality of Psalm 23: "Yea, though I walk through the valley of the shadow of death, I will fear no evil, for you are with me." I don't have to be afraid. Words like "palliative" don't exactly conjure up warm fuzzies, but I know that this hurting is for such a short time…and what waits for me is a forever that is so much more beautiful than even the prettiest cherry blossoms. He is worthy, friends. Oh, He is worthy. This Thanksgiving season, when on the surface it may look so dark, I will still be grateful. He has given me so much—SO MUCH—that I don't deserve. Jesus owes me nothing, yet He gave everything. Me and my wiffle ball-sized Monster will worship and give thanks. He is good all the time. THAT is TRUTH. P.S. My grandparents love me a lot. Like, a bushel and a peck. At age 38, that still amazes me, and is one of the most precious things I know in this life.

Digging Out

Thursday, December 12, 2013

Six Days. Six Days. SIX DAYS!

Six days is how long it has been since we have had any kind of normal (cough, cough) in our household. Six days ago, Old Man Winter caught DFW in his sights, and life as we know it came to a complete standstill. Here's what I've learned in the last almost-week:

Ice is pretty when it blankets your world and you can snuggle up by the fire with nowhere to go. Ice is fun when school is cancelled for the first day. Ice ceases to be pretty or fun when school keeps closing and cabin fever sets in. If you live in a continual state of winter, 3 pairs of flannel pajamas is not enough. A major ice storm is in Texas what a major heat wave is in New York. You can only toss so many coats, jeans, gloves, scarves, hats, and socks in the dryer at one time. Little boys do not freeze or tire easily. You should clear the ice not only from your windshield, but also from the roof of your vehicle before you drive.

Our children's children will be regaling their children with stories of The Great Ice Storm of 2013. How we didn't see our youngest for more than 24 hours because he went to a friend's house and stayed…and stayed…and stayed. Or how we got what seemed to be the last loaf of bread in the city before store shelves were completely emptied by crazy frantic citizens…or how the freighbor girls, who hail from Michigan, shared their real live sled and showed our Texas boys a thing or two.

Finally—FINALLY!—this morning, everyone went back to work and school. I love my family, but all of this quality time (and wet shoes tracking in leaves and mud) has pushed all of us a little closer than we want to be. There is still plenty of ice around. We live on the north/sunny side of our street and there are still several inches on our back patio! Across the street, where there are more shadows than sun, dangerous icicles (seriously!) still hang from the rooftops and the sheet of white in the yards remains largely the same. Every night, what little bit has melted refreezes on the driveways and sidewalks. Because it's still cold. Yesterday we reached a whopping 37 degrees…heat wave!!!!

Now, you might be wondering how a Texas girl passes the time when she is iced in. Good question. I'll tell you: She warms up with a bit of radiation. Oh, yes. While the rest of the world is snuggled up drinking hot coca and playing board games, I (and my darling I'll-do-anything-for-you friend, Rachel), drove into Dallas to the hospital for radiation treatments.

Here's the deal on radiation: I've never done it before. I've never done it before because radiation is not a typical treatment for ovca patients. In my case, the cancer has been too widespread to risk radiation in lieu of more traditional treatments. Now, though, I've exhausted traditional. We are all done with standard. The choices are 1) Non-traditional, or 2) Nothing. So, I am allowing myself to be radiated. In exchange for making the trip to the hospital every. single. day., (You heard me. Monday through Friday, for three weeks. I get off on Christmas Eve and Christmas Day.) allowing strangers to use me for their own personal sketchbooks ("x" marks the spot!), and risking a slew of side effects (they were said to be no big deal. Liars.), I might get some relief from the harsh, relentless symptoms of fast-growing Monster. Did I make a deal with the devil? Perhaps. It has not been an easy go. Of course, everything that could go wrong, has gone wrong. Topping the list: nausea, extreme fatigue, and fever-like chills and shivers. Rounding out my bottom-of-the-barrel, my radiation oncologist had a medical emergency of his own and will be out for the remainder of the month.

Reeeaaalllyyy?!? I only need him this month.

This morning I woke up feeling super-nauseous. I have plenty of meds to meet all sorts of needs, but today not even prescription-strength anti-nausea was making dents. I went ahead and went to radiation anyway, because I thought I could not feel much yuckier.

Bad call. I found out I could feel worse, and I found it out while I was getting sick in a McDonald's parking lot close to Highway 75, with my deserves-better-than-me freighbor patting my back and looking on helplessly. (I switched drivers yesterday. Lucky Rachel.)

Damn cancer.

I hate this wretched disease. If you piled all of my "dislikes" together—cold feet, wet blue jeans, empty toilet paper rolls, children with no manners, alarm clocks—it still could not amount to the level of hatred I have for cancer.

Susan graciously delivered me into my own driveway, although hers is about 10 feet away. I managed to wiggle back in to my pjs and when Little Middle and Baby got off the bus, they found me on the couch in exactly the same position I was in when they went to school this morning.

I've had a few words to say to God about this new treatment, and they haven't all been nice. Actually, hardly any of them have been nice! I am so over it.

When I started writing this post this morning from my position on the sofa, I occasionally glanced up to look at this:

It's not a perfect tree, but it's ours. There is something really peaceful about sitting by the Christmas tree, isn't there? I yearn for that peace all the time. It is a hard-fought battle every day. "Let every heart prepare Him room…"

Lord, please help me to make room for you. Thank you for being my Friend and for being a safe place for me to go. Please give me joy, especially in this season. I want to be soft and open to You and to Your spirit. I believe that you can heal, both inside and out.

Please let this be a season of healing and miracles. I want to be ready to receive my King: You. Thank you for loving me and for your promises that are always true. Amen.

All I Can Say

Saturday, January 11, 2014

Lord, I'm tired.

I have fought this Monster for a long time. Seven years. Nearly the entirety of my Baby's life. I have had surgeries. I've been hospitalized multiple times. I have done chemotherapy… five times. I lost my hair, my eyebrows, and my eyelashes. I've given up my dignity and my spirit has been crushed. I endured radiation as long as I could. My skin has been burnt to a crisp. I've traveled the country, made countless appointments, and researched until my eyes were crossed.

Lord, I'm so alone.

No one understands—really understands—what it feels like to be me. I have an army of friends and family who have walked with me and stood in the gap for me. But nobody fully can understand the fear of laying on that CT scan table over and over again, month after month, year after year. No one else can really identify with that feeling I get in my stomach while I wait for the phone to ring with news—that is always bad. No one sees the way people look at me with pity or worse, look at my children. No one but me can read the precious cards that come in the mail that all say, "I am praying for healing,"…and then wonder why God isn't answering that prayer.

Lord, the dark is creeping in, it's creeping up to swallow me. God and I, we've stayed up a lot of nights together. Seven years equals a lot of insomnia. There have been nights where I've cried, nights where I've begged, and nights when I've tried to ignore Him altogether. (That never worked out great for me.) We've had days, when I've been alone in bed, and I could literally feel the disease—the darkness—moving closer.

I think I'll stop, rest here awhile. I had an appointment with Dr. F this week. I was very clear as I explained to him how I have been suffering. I told him how radiation has made me SO UNBELIEVABLY SICK, and how I feel like I made a deal with the devil by agreeing to do it. I am weak, and crazy tired. I calmly listed out the symptoms I am experiencing, and then sat back, swiped at the frustrated tears falling down my cheeks, and listened as my entire life changed…again. It is time, he said. And this is all that I can say right now. I am sick because of the progression of the disease. I have used up all of the treatment options, and there is simply nothing else to do. He is recommending that we start looking at hospice. He doesn't suggest that for patients unless he can estimate that the remaining time left to live is six months (or less). Lord, didn't you see me crying? I was barely aware of the tears that persistently fell. I hung on every word that Nurse Allyson spoke about hospice: where to look, what to ask about, how it works. I nearly missed my sweet Dr. F, out of the corner of my eye, reach for the Kleenex box. It took me a moment to figure out that he was crying, too.

And didn't you hear me call your name? It ended with Dr. F just asking me to let him know what I decide. When I give the green light, he and Nurse Allyson will go to the ends of the earth to help me find the right people, get the right meds, and be as comfortable as possible. They both hugged me, and I walked out of there, stunned. Of course, nothing that he said was a real surprise. I think I felt it in my body long before I heard the words. There is simply a bit of shock value to hearing someone verbalize such absolutes. Wasn't it you I gave my heart to? Six months. Or less. I wish you'd remember where you sat it down. There is still the idea of the clinical trial at MD Anderson. It is Dr. F's belief (and I have no reason to doubt him) that the trial would not result in any significant extension or quality of life for me. There are decisions to make. Many hard decisions. And this is all that I can say right now. And this is all that I can give. And this is all that I can say right now, And this is all that I can give, that's my everything. I've walked with Jesus for a long, long time. I don't claim to know everything, or to understand why he does what he does. Not by a long shot. As the darkness creeps closer, I have to dig deep to get back to what I do know is Truth: 1) God loves me. 2) God will take care of me. 3) God is always in control. These are The Three Things that I have taught my boys. The four of us have recited them over and over again until we were red in the face and they were rolling their eyes at me. But The Three Things have never been more important than they are now. This is all that I can say right now. "Yet I am always with you; you hold me by my right hand. You guide me with your counsel, and afterward you will take me into glory. Whom have I in heaven but you? And earth has nothing I desire besides you. My flesh and my heart may fail, but God is the strength of my heart and my portion forever." Psalm 73:23–26

Yes, that's my everything.

Not Forgotten

Friday, January 17, 2014

Life for the past 9 days has been a crazy roller coaster ride. I alternate between bouts of tears and moments of peace. I have done my best to balance my need to be with friends and loved ones with my almost insatiable desire to be alone. I have read my Bible and I have heaved huge, you-don't-know-what-you're-doing sighs at God. I have laid in bed and I have gone to Target. I have also done quite a bit of worrying. It wasn't too many weeks ago that I told you that my husband had lost his job. Truth be told, it was a terrible way to end a terrible year…and a terrifying way to begin a new one. I suppose it goes without saying that we need him to be working. Insurance alone is absolutely necessary (and crazy expensive). He is looking. He has made some contacts, and had a few interviews. So far, though, nothing too solid or promising has come his way. We paid the January bills, and then we started crunching numbers. Every which way we trimmed it, there were more bills than money. And so I worried. I despaired. I fretted. And yesterday, I threw a pity party for one: ME. I sat on my comfy bed in my warm house in my clean, soft pajamas, and I used my computer to read about hospice services. And I cried.

Three Little Cowboys

Goodness, did I cry! Finally, after a couple of hours, I slammed my laptop shut and I said to God only three words: "Where. Are. You.?????" This afternoon, Baby brought in the mail. He likes to sort it into five piles: Hubby, Me, Goliath, Little Middle, and his own. (Today, his and Goliath's piles were empty, but Little Middle scored a hunting magazine!) When he ran back outside to play, I went through the stacks again. Bill, bill, W-2, advertisement, sweet card, sweet card, more bills...and an envelope. Curiosity got the best of me and I opened it. Inside that ordinary-looking envelope was a check. Are you sitting down, friend? It was a check payable to Hubby for the exact amount that we need to make our next mortgage and insurance payments. THE EXACT AMOUNT. To the dollar, what we had discussed and agreed that we need. God was there. He has been working, even as I have worried. We are not forgotten. I collapsed into a chair, and with fresh tears streaming down my cheeks, I called my husband. I told him, and he simply said, "Praise God." Friends, we do not know where the money came from. All we know is that our very real God met our very real need with a miracle in the mail. Isn't that just like our Lord? To show up in an unexpected, unusual way to prove that his promises are 100% true? So many things remain unknowns in my life. There are inquiries to be made and caregiver interviews to be conducted. There are details to be attended to and decisions to be made. There are unthinkable conversations to be held with my three little cowboys. But my question from yesterday has been answered : "Never will I leave you; never will I forsake you." (Hebrews 13:5) I still have goose bumps on my arms, and I'm sniffly from crying. But my heart...oh, my heart is refreshed. No doubt that could have happened without such a blatant miracle. I am so incredibly thankful. Thankful for the miracle in the mail...thankful that I belong to a God who loves and provides...thankful that I am never beyond his reach or outside of his care. We are not forgotten.

Allyson Hendrickson

> Are not five sparrows sold for two pennies? Yet not one of them is forgotten by God. Indeed, the very hairs of your head are all numbered. Don't be afraid; you are worth more than many sparrows. (Luke 12:6–7)

Sovereign

Wednesday, January 29, 2014

Good news first: Hubby has a job! There is a whole back story of an interview, a staffing recruiter who dropped the ball, a prayer time where the two of us petitioned the Lord and honestly poured out our hurting hearts, and then a whirlwind 24 hours of contacts and circumstances that only our good, never-lets-go God could have orchestrated. He starts on Monday. His first paycheck will come in at just about the time we expect that the "reserves" will run out. Huh. Just in telling you that mini-story, there is light shining through the darkness that has been this day. I actually intended to pour out my sad, hurting heart again here to you this afternoon. I meant to tell you about pain that refuses to be managed and the gray, Eeyore-ish cloud that was above my head when I woke up this morning. I wanted to tell you that I cancelled a coffee date with a friend and I have let my phone go to voice mail because I simply couldn't get past myself. I intended to tell you that I haven't even changed out of my pajamas today, and if I were to be really honest, I would have confessed that I could not wait until the cowboys left for school this morning so I could get on with the business of feeling sorry for myself. Deep breath. I flipped open my laptop to do just that, and Hubby said, "Oh—are you going to write about the job?" I didn't tell him that his brand new, answer-to-many-prayers job wasn't even on my radar. I simply replied, "Of course!"…and I acted as if that had been my intention the entire time. Huh. It's a weird thing about being diagnosed with a terminal illness…your perspective changes almost instantly. I'm not talking even about the initial diagnosis. For seven years now, I have had some treatment up my sleeve. There has been a "next thing," something else to try—some reason to believe that certainly, surely there was no way that God was going to let me die. No, it's the part where there is no more medicine or technology or earthly intervention that can fix it. The part where the doctor looks you straight in the eye and says, "I'm sorry. There is nothing else to do." I've always seen the world through pretty black-and-white lenses. It's one of the best things about me, and it can also be one of the worst things about me. But now, almost overnight, my perspective has been even more narrowed. I just want to get straight to the bottom line. Only a few things really matter, quite a lot of other things don't matter much at all. People matter. Families matter. Time matters. Jesus matters. It's also super-easy to forget the things that matter and to self-focus. It is, after all, ME who is sick. I am the one who has to deal with stuff no one my age should have to think about: hospice services, wills and other legal documents, funeral arrangements. Sometimes my pain can be managed, other times it is unbearable. Nearly everything I do requires hard work: showering, helping with 4th grade fractions, explaining my decisions/feelings to everyone. My life has been turned upside down by this wretched Sickness. (Quick story: When Goliath was three, Seester and I had a garage sale at our parents' house. While we were working ourselves to death in the Houston hellish inferno weather, Goliath and Abby Dog were watching us from a window. Thus, my small son witnessed the patrons who wheeled his tiny bicycle out of my parents' garage and tried to buy it from us. His comment to his Nana: "Those are wretched, wretched people!" That is how 'wretched' came to be one of my very favorite words of all time.) "These are uphill, into-the-wind challenges you are facing. They are not easy. But neither are they random. God is not sometimes sovereign. He is not occasionally victorious. He does not occupy the throne one day and vacate it the next. "The Lord shall not turn back until He has executed and accomplished the thoughts and intents of His mind" (Jeremiah 30:24).

> "This season in which you find yourself may puzzle you, but it does not bewilder God. He can and will use it for his purpose."
>
> —Max Lucado, *You'll Get Through This*

It's not about me at all. Some days, like today, I need to breathe deeply and take a few steps back in order to get a clear picture. This Sickness—this life—is not at all what I thought it would be. I didn't plan on this or want this or even see it coming. But my uprooted plans and my changing circumstances do not change who God is. Not one little bit. He remains the same, whether I have a "good" day and I feel like my old self, or a bad day, and I barely manage to brush my teeth. (Hmmm…did I brush my teeth this morning?) He is sovereign. He is good. He intends great things for me, and he is determined to see them through to completion. There is comfort in that for me.

Truth be told, I've hated this day. It's dark out now, and I will be glad to go to sleep and put it behind me. Tomorrow, my new hospice nurse is making her first official visit. I'm not sure I'm exactly looking forward to that either, but I am certain that my Jesus has already gone ahead and paved the way. Just as he made provision for Hubby's new job, he will take care of this new chapter of the journey.

Don't you wonder how people who don't have Jesus get through life? I think about that all the time. My darkest days are

Allyson Hendrickson

still lined with victory. I hope that you know him, friend. I am so grateful that I can have hope to fall back on when the days are overwhelming. I'm so thankful that all the pieces of my life are in his hands. Tomorrow is a new day. Great is his faithfulness.

The Day I Told Them the Truth

Friday, February 07, 2014

Dear Cowboys,

I feel like although I desperately want to forget it ever happened, I need to commemorate in a small way the Day I Told You The Truth. One minute, we were a regular family of five playing a board game. The next minute, we were a group of broken-hearted people. The game lay forgotten for hours, until I pulled myself together enough to clean it up. I don't think we'll be pulling it out to play for quite a while. There is really no good way to break terrible news to the people you love the most. I struggled for days with what to say to you, and all I could really think was, "This is so unfair. This is so unfair." Every interaction with you became all the more precious, because I knew that you were walking around in a bubble, of sorts. A bubble where your little world was intact and safe...a bubble that I was going to burst.

And burst it I did! I'm so sorry, heart boys. I'm so very sorry that we live in a world that is not fair. I'm so sorry that after all this time and effort, I haven't been able to beat this thing. I'm sorry that I can't stay with you. I'm sorry that I couldn't protect you.

I will never forget your blank looks. I was telling you the awful truth, but doing my best to avoid using scary words. I don't know if you really did not understand, or if you just didn't want to know. Whatever it was, I knew I had to be straightforward. So I started saying things like "not much longer," "dying," and "not going to get well." It felt like plunging into a freezing cold body of water. I couldn't seem to get enough air, and there was no way to go back and undo the huge jump I had taken.

Oh, loves. Your sweet faces were almost too much. I wanted to reach out and touch you…hug you…comfort you, but there was no room for that. The closer I moved to you, the farther you moved away from me. It was almost as if my physical presence was too much for you One of you moved to Daddy's lap. One of you continued to stare at me, as if you didn't even know me. One of you got up and simply walked out of the house. I expected different reactions from each of you, as God made you so wonderfully different. I was not prepared for such dramatic responses.

In a weird way, I was touched. Your strong reactions definitely showed me that you love me. The news I was delivering was not easy, and you demonstrated that you were hurting. I a m crazy-thankful for the intense feelings you have for your mama, because they mean that I matter. The Monster has had a way of making me feel inferior in the worst ways, but you three never fail to bring out my best.

I guess that's the key. There is no doubt that I was created for this. There are lots of other things I do, people I know, places I go, identities I have in this life. But all of them pale in comparison to being your mom. There is nothing else I want to do. Being your mom makes me a better person.

We will make it through this, my sons. I hate—HATE!!!—that you are suffering because of me. Because of my sickness. Not a single days goes by that I don't pray for physical healing so you can have the mom you deserve to have. Not one night do I fall asleep before I've begged God to guard your hearts and pave your ways. Not one.

As hard as it is to understand (I don't fully understand it myself), I want you to KNOW beyond a shadow of a doubt that God is good. I do not believe that God caused my cancer, but he did allow it. He is still good, and He loves you even more than I do. Cling to that truth with all that you have, babies. I am.

And let's hold on to one another. Whatever time I have left to be with you, I want to be meaningful time. I want to soak up every delicious minute of laughing with (and at) you. I want to create beautiful memories for you, even if we have to hurry up and squeeze all of those memories into a short time period. Let's do it. Let's live big and love bigger. I already love you all so much.

With my whole heart, Mom

Limitations

Thursday, February 20, 2014

THIS IS A WEIRD TIME in my life. I've tried to think of other, better words. Lonely. Scary. Sad. Weird. I am working on creating—and accepting—a new normal for myself. This week, I've resigned from one of my last just-for-me activities, a volunteer position at Goliath's middle school. I simply don't have the energy or the physical stamina, to go and push buttons on a copy machine. It's really unbelievable to me.

    I feel a little lost. I feel easily replaceable. It truly stuns me when I go out during the day and I see the little old man down the street preparing the soil in his gardens for the spring planting. Or when I hear the stories from my friends of what they've been up to, or notice the neighbors coming and going while I sit in the front room. Really…I don't expect that the world will continue to go like it always does—because I'm not in it. My husband is slowly but steadily taking over a lot of my stuff at home. My mom, and this week my dad, has been here taking care of me and doing a lot of the work. My darling housekeeper is even coming two days a week instead of her usual one Tuesday to help out.

Three Little Cowboys

While I am so appreciative of these people who love me and are helping with the transition process for my cowboys, my old self wants to jump up and do it all—just because it is mine to do. I want my mom to have her life back, my husband to just go to work and leave the running and the scheduling and the cooking to me, and I want Amparo to...well, I honestly don't mind her coming twice a week. I've finally found the solution to the laundry problem!!!

Mostly, I want my life back. I'm not angry or anything. Just sad. Because I had this great world made out of kids and noise and food and preschool and friends and shopping and taking care of things and church and activity and sharing and being a part of people. I mattered. And it was meaningful and sometimes messy, but wonderfully beautiful life. Now I have...what? A good bed and a quiet room and a few pairs of pajamas that I wear all the time. It pales in comparison.

A friend posted these words on Facebook last week from Jesus Calling:

"Thank Me for the conditions that are requiring you to be still...Instead of resenting the limitations of a weakened body, search for My way in the midst of those very circumstances. Limitations can be liberating when your strongest desire is living close to Me...My strength and power show themselves most effective in weakness."

The day I read that, I wrote this in my journal:

"It's hard to be thankful for these conditions. I overdid it yesterday, and I paid for it today. It's so frustrating! Why can't I have at least a semi-regular life where I can do at least a few normal things? Can my limitations really be liberating??? Strong word. Oh, for grace to trust Him more!"

I want to be thankful. I really do. Being still is hard. Being weak is harder. I know God is in this new chapter. But the quieter it gets, the harder it is to hear Him.

Oh, for grace to trust Him more.

Living with Grace

Wednesday, February 26, 2014

It is a struggle, as I sit down to write this evening, to form all of my thoughts into a cohesive format. This day...oh, my.

It started as a regular day with regular cinnamon toast. Then Nurse came. Ten minutes into her visit, I knew I was going to throw up, and promptly did so. Maybe I have not made it clear here before, so I will do it now: I hate vomiting. It's for sure in my top 3 things I despise. Right after I returned from brushing my teeth, Nurse re-introduced the prospects of "assistance equipment," including an oxygen tank and a wheelchair. She first introduced the ideas during her visits last week, when I quickly and distinctly turned her down.

I lost the battle today. I am now the horrified owner of a WHEELCHAIR, which you will NEVER see me in.

She left, and then I threw up twice more. THEN, my sweet Goliath came to me to confess that he "accidentally" read something on my iPad that was hurtful to me, so it was also hurtful to him. He was full of questions and a little bit angry. That caused me to ask more questions and be a little a lot angry all over again. Stupid day. What I really want to do here, though, is tell you about last night. This conversation happened: Goliath: So Mom, you know how you have that cancer? Me: Yes. Yes, I do. G: Well, I need to talk to you about something. I'm not sure if it's wrong or not, though. Me: You can tell me anything, buddy. G: You know I would do anything for you, right? Me: Yeah... G: Every night when I go to bed and I say my bedtime prayers, I pray for you to not have to have cancer anymore. And a lot of nights, I pray that God would just give me your cancer instead. You know, so I could be sick instead of you. Me: (Solid, streaming tears) G: Is it wrong for me to pray that, Mom? I think at that very moment I understood for the first time how sad my parents must be. Because the very thought of my baby having to go through this horrible, wretched disease made my head spin and my heart nearly split in two. At the very thought. I somehow managed to keep my head on and I dried up my tears. I told my precious baby boy how God doesn't want bad things to happen to us, but they do because we do not live in a perfect world. I reminded him how God wanted perfection for us (remember the Garden of Eden?), but sin messed that all up. I said to him that God has a good plan and great ideas for all of us, and as Christ-followers, one of the hardest things we have to do sometimes is to BELIEVE that is true and TRUST Him to see it through. Yes, even if our mom has cancer. Yes, even if it turns our lives upside down. Yes, even if it sucks. (I allow this boy 'o mine to say the word "sucks" only when it is used in combination with the word "cancer." True mom story.) Then I said to Goliath that while I don't think he's necessarily wrong to pray this particular prayer, that I wish he wouldn't do it anymore. Simply because I can't stand the thought that God could choose to answer his prayer. No more than I can believe that I gave birth to a person who would do anything for me. He's only twelve—and I totally believe he would do it if he could. Grace is getting something you totally don't deserve...and if being this kid's mom isn't grace, I don't know what is.

Bellies, Beds, and Body Bags

Friday, March 14, 2014

I have a Monster growing inside of me. There is no denying his existence, nor his growth. Yesterday, I looked like myself. A little rough, yes, because I was in dire need of a good hair-washing and some fresh pajamas. But other than that, I looked like me. This morning I got up and I look like me…at 5-months pregnant! Seriously. I called Nurse in a bit of a frenzied panic. How could this happen just…overnight?!? She calmly told me a story about abdominal disease and fluid build-up. I not-so-calmly asked her what we could do about it. Her answer? Nothing. That's what. We do NOTHING about so much accumulation of fluid that I look like my former pregnant self. Wha…??? This just keeps getting better.

Then, I went on a little field trip with Hubby and Daddy. We went to a funeral home. I'd been there before, when my friend lost her own daddy in a sad and sudden way. I had no real emotion going in. Actually, I felt a little detached. Maybe that's why I was so surprised to see a dead person first thing upon entry. She was just laying there in a room off to the side, surrounded by floral sprays, waiting for her friends and family to come pay their respects. I actually whispered out loud, "There's a dead person over there." Stating the obvious didn't help, but it broke the ice when the funeral director came out at that exact moment.

He seated us in a conference room that was not spectacular by any means. I could have been at any company in Anytown, USA. This room was only set apart by the collection of urns in a glass case in the corner. The Director took a seat at the head of the table and started his spiel. He did a good job. We were well-armed with a list of questions and ideas, and Mr. Director provided all the answers that we needed. He also gave us some good information about cemeteries in the area. Since I am lacking in this area of expertise, I felt grateful. Did you know that not all cemeteries have perpetual care? If you are a local, this might explain a lot to you like it did for me.

I never realized how many decisions there are to make for a funeral. I have been working on a few things on my own at home, but WOW! Who knew? One of the most important decisions to make is the choosing of the casket. We were quickly educated about the differences in steel grades, wood types, and then we were allowed to enter The Casket Room. It wasn't like the casket rooms that you see on TV and such. There were only 8 full-size caskets in the room. The rest of the displays were just cut pieces of the casket with a pull-out display from the wall. Weird, but efficient.

I found one I liked. I mean, I guess I like it. Again, weird. Mr. Director regaled us with a tale of a husband and wife who visited The Casket Room and asked him to take their pictures inside their caskets of choice. Why? What in the world is wrong with people?!? I guess that's one way you can really be sure you're getting what you like.

While I held up pretty well through the funeral home experience, I must confess that I am a little freaked out by the thought of bugs and creepy-crawlies and, um, elements getting through. Hence the need for an outer burial container, but still…

ew. That's the only thing that really bothered me. I was pretty calm as Mr. Director went down the list of his a la carte menu. We selected some things we really wanted, and drew question marks beside others that require decisions. Then we thanked him for his time and went on our way.

For as much as I had been dreading this visit, I suppose it went relatively well. I did it, and I'm proud of myself for that. I feel like taking care of these things is a way that I can take care of my family. They don't need to see to all these little details and worries if I can do it for them while I'm still here.

Right now I am waiting for Nurse to come. This will be the third appearance she has made at my house this week. Maybe it's just me, but I'm thinking a 3/5 ratio of nurse needs isn't that great. She's coming to access my port (which I haven't used since last spring—almost one year). They are going to "feed" me some of my medications through my port so I have fewer pills to take. It's a lovely thought, because I have got some pills!

Mom bought me one of those old-people pill organizers. It's the supreme version:

Nifty, huh? Every one of those little spaces is filled up with pills for me to take. Every. Single. Day. It's a lot.

Update: Nurse has come and gone. She totally threw me under the bus to Hubby and Daddy about not wanting to use the wheelchair. Which I don't. I was thinking maybe we could take it when we go to look at cemeteries. Seems appropriate. She managed to access the port with minimal discomfort to me. I am most thankful. The port has always been a difficult thing to deal with. Maybe now I know that the medical staff just weren't doing it right!

I now am receiving methadone through the mediport. I am hooked up to it, which means I must carry it with me all the time, everywhere I go. Ugh...I hate that. Just looking at the unattractive bag which houses it, I am already freaking out, wondering how I will carry it around and what I can possibly wear that will hide the tube sticking out of my chest (and disguise my giant belly). Again: ugh. These are problems I didn't sign up for when Monster came nosing around.

Also, this afternoon we are expecting delivery of a hospital bed. Nurse asked me how I had been sleeping, and the answer is, "Not well." I even take Ambien, the magic med, every night, and I am still waking up several times each night because I am crazy uncomfortable. It's like she can read my mind. Nurse said that is due to the swelling in my abdomen, and that laying flat will become increasingly difficult. Then she gently reminded me that I could have a hospital bed that can elevate my head and/or feet, and it would probably be a great time for it. I agreed, even though it's about the last thing in the world I want to have in my possession (except a wheelchair). So there is one coming. I think that the only twin sheets we have left are Goliath's old ones with the camo pattern. Mom suggested that I send Daddy to Target to buy pretty new ones for my "new" bed. Or maybe I'll just sleep on the camo sheets for a few days.

P.S. Just in case you ever need to know, "disaster pouch" is a nice way of saying "body bag."

Ally's Wish

Monday, March 31, 2014

CANCER IS A LONELY PLACE to be. Instead of planning out dinner menus and baseball schedules, I'm making end-of-life plans. Instead of dreaming up the next family vacation, I'm fretting over life insurance policies and trust funds for the boys.

I have good people in my life. Really. I have GOOD people in my life. A few weeks ago, I met a group of friends for dinner. I had no idea why we were gathered, but I quickly found out that it wasn't just to talk about hedgehogs, our kids, and shampoo. No, they had something much bigger and more important. Something that made me forget for a while that my life is not what I want it to be:

Ally's Wish is a new foundation put together by my amazing friends. The purpose of Ally's Wish is to grant wishes for other mothers with terminal illness. Spread joy. Give hope!

I can not think of a more fantastic way for my legacy to live on. It's not often that I am without words, but I was at the dinner table that night. My friend Missy explained to me how she had been praying faithfully for me (which I knew she had been). Like so many of us, she wanted to do something. She wanted to put something behind her words. But she didn't know what. So… she kept praying. And one morning, God gave it to her. She immediately called the other friends, and Ally's Wish was born. They had the whole thing put together and finished before they ever even presented it to me. There was not a fear that I would say "no." Because God was at work…there was something so much bigger happening than what any of us could ever do on our own.

At dinner that night, they asked me what my wish is. They wanted mine to be the first one granted. They said that I should dream big. They said that I should think outside the box. They said that I am loved, and that people want to help.

So, I am thrilled to tell you that my wish is for this blog to be published. I don't necessarily want it to be on a shelf in every Barnes & Noble across America, but I want it to be published at least so that each of my boys can have a copy of their own—a way for them to remember that their mom loved them with every inch of her heart.

Maybe you want to help. Maybe God is leading you to bring hope to other sick mothers the way these friends of mine have brought hope to me. Maybe you want to donate or volunteer. Go to our website and look around. I hope your heart is touched and you are moved to help. On behalf of moms like me who love their kids and will have to leave them sooner than we want to…thank you. Thank you for being an instrument in God's hands. Thank you for reminding us that there are still good things to be had, joy to fill hearts like ours. He is a good God.

Catching Up

April 13, 2014

THE GOOD NEWS NEVER STOPS. My computer died. Apparently, according to my IT-gifted Hubby who is supper amazing and I have not said enough about through this ordeal, it was a tragic, nothing-could-have-stopped-it death. Irreversible. Bad news for someone who passes many of the hours of the day online. He has been there with me through the roughest parts from the beginning and to even blog about it is too hard.

Sigh.

The computer I'm using now is one that Hubs managed to resurrect "just enough" from the family electronic graveyard (What? Doesn't your family have one of those?!?). He pulled a power cord from the mix-and-match pile that fortuitously made the green light come on. Ahhh…sweet relief!

Baby has taken a liking to Goliath's euphonium. 90% of the time, Goliath fails to put the instrument fully away in its case, which is more of a temptation than his youngest brother can handle. I doubt I will ever fully get used to that which sounds like a dying animal in my front room.

Little Middle is playing baseball for the first time. Unless you are a baseball mom, you can NOT understand the feeling of the knot in the pit of your stomach when your little guy steps up to bat. No amount of time spent in the batting cages or balls tossed in the backyard can prepare either one of you for the enormous pressure of wanting needing to make the aluminum 'POP!' sound when the bat and ball make contact. The pressure is SO intense, in fact, that when the pitcher (whose mother is biting her fingernails 2 rows in front of you, by the way) pegs your little man with the ball on his fifth pitch, you have to restrain yourself from rushing the mound to hug him because your kid just walked to 1st base!!! And so it goes…until the next time he goes up to bat. There is not enough Xanax on the planet for this wonderful walk into the world of beginning baseball.

Of course, real life continues to barrel its way straight through our family. Kids can say and do the darndest things, but Monster threatens to cover their light with his darkness. Truthfully, each morning I open my eyes, and I am disappointed. What I would really like to have happen is that I could go to heaven one night while I sleep. Wouldn't that be perfectly lovely? Fall asleep and transition from this stupid broken world into the next beautifully perfect one. Talk about a dream come true!

I have "settled" (a term I use super-loosely) into a daily sick routine. I still get up and wake the boys up at their appointed times each morning. This is my favorite. I think, especially for the littles, that it helps promote a sense of normalcy, i.e. "Mom's face is the first one I see in the morning. That is right." We get them fed, dressed, and out the door, usually on time, with lunches in their hands and completed homework in their backpacks.

I know that's a lot more than what a lot of healthy parents are able to do, so I try to be thankful. Honestly, though, it's not enough for me. I can't believe that I, who was once such a hands-on, do-it-all mom, have been reduced to a watch-themshov-el-in-Lucky-Charms mom who considers it a successful morning if she doesn't vomit in front of them.

After they go to school, I breathe a sigh of relief, take my first handful of many pills, and make my first big decision of the day: to shower or bathe? Yes, I do one of the other each day. Both are wrought with perils that an ordinary person might not consider. A shower means that I need to wash my hair, a problem all in itself. Fortunately, I have added to my repertoire of medical equipment a shower chair. I hate it just like I hate all the other stuff. BUT... you'd be surprised how helpful it has been in doing something as simple as washing my hair. I had one morning when my sweet daddy was here that I asked him to help me wash my hair over the kitchen sink. It was the day after that that the shower chair was delivered! A bath...well, who doesn't like a nice warm bath every now and then? Especially when they don't feel well? The problem with that is that I keep falling asleep in the bathtub. It's happened so often that now my caretakers (i.e. Hubby and Mom) have strict instructions from Nurse to keep a close eye on me. That eye that she has in mind is closer than I will allow, so we've had to compromise with sponge baths a few times.

After I get cleaned up and changed into fresh pj's, it's time for a nap. Yes, even though I just got up, it's time to go back to bed. Very often, I will sleep for another 2 hours (or longer). Truthfully, I wish my body would allow me to sleep even longer. There are points in the day that I think would be better if I just let go and slept straight through.

When I wake up, sometimes I eat lunch, and sometimes I eat nothing at all. It all depends on how I'm feeling. I can't seem to hold interest in my books. I've always been an avid reader! But right now, for example, I am at the halfway point in a new book by one of my favorite authors, and I just can't feign enough interest to talk myself into reading further. What a letdown. I'm not much of a TV or movie person, but a lot of times I leave it on for background noise. What else am I going to do?

I don't drive anymore. Correction: I can drive, but I don't. I am taking so much medication (23 pills a day to be exact, and that's without "extra" stuff like phenergran for nausea or Xanax for my 6th grader stress), that who knows what is happening to my response times, my reflexes, etc. So I depend on Hubby or the occasional friend to get me where I need to go. It's not really that hard to work out, because I don't leave the house much. Still, the loss of that independence stings. It's amazing how I never seemed to care about just getting out of the house for no reason before, and now that I can't, it really feels like it matters. The Bus just sits in the driveway, seemingly taunting me.

Anyway, back to the rundown of my day: The boys come home in the afternoon, and then the craziest thing happens. I swear that as soon as the door opens and I hear the first, "Hi, Mom!," my stomach starts to hurt. I become uncomfortable in my own skin, and that horrible feeling increases over the next several hours until the clock mercifully allows me to take bedtime meds and I can sleep. I don't know why those two things have to intersect, but that is what happens nearly every. single. day. I hate it so much, because I feel like I don't spend nearly the time with them that I want to. They come in my room and tell me about their day, of course, but I'm no match for them. Most nights I have reading time with Baby, usually some math or some other can't-wait-to-be-done assignment with Little Middle, and then Goliath will come in and demonstrate his newest playlist for me before bedtime. I am so thankful for these times with them, but again: it's not enough. I've fallen hard. And every day is a tough reminder that I'm not what I used to be.

So that's a typical day. Of course, weekends are a little different. I have been trying very hard to make Little Middle's baseball and Baby's soccer games. Hubby and I sat out in the crazy wind on Saturday morning cheering for a bunch of second graders who were falling all over themselves. Hilarious! But even that felt bad to me: I used to be the team mom. I went to every practice, I set up the snack schedule, I made sure he had his cleats, his socks, his shin guards for every practice and game. Now I have no idea how it all comes together each week! Of course, I'm not so arrogant as to believe that the world of soccer needs me to make it all jive. I simply miss being an integral part of my children's lives. And I'm at a loss how to achieve that feeling of closeness again in this new world.

The boys seem to be doing well. They have each had their own mini-breakdowns from time to time, and that is to be expected. I don't think you live knowing that your mother is dying and not have issues. School teachers, counselors, coaches, church personnel…they're all on board with us. There are people falling over themselves waiting and wanting to help the 3 little cowboys. And for that, ya'll, I am unbelievably, overwhelmingly thankful. Crazy thankful. God has been so gracious to put our family in a place where we are cared for and loved on. There's no way that the boys could be carrying on so well if they weren't in the middle of a you-are-loved cloud everywhere they go. Life is hard enough, and a curveball like this can really alter the course of one's entire life one way or the other if we let it.

I still worry, of course. I spend a lot of those empty hours in my days worrying. Some days I feel like all I DO is worry. I love this translation of a well-known verse: "Don't fret or worry. Instead of worrying, pray. Let petitions and praises shape your worries into prayers, letting God know your concerns. Before you know it, a sense of God's whole-ness, everything coming together for good, will come and settle you down. It's wonderful what happens when Christ displaces worry at the center of your life." (Philippians 4:6–7, MSG) This Scripture offers an option: Instead of worrying, pray. And don't just pray asking for things, but offer up praise. I love that. If I am doing it right, I shouldn't just ask God for his watchcare over my sons. I should praise Him! And there's plenty to praise Him for: He is big enough to handle my requests. He loves the boys even more than I love them. He has good plans for them. And before I know it, my need to worry is replaced with Christ. A sense of God's wholeness…I can't think of anything better to have on this earth until I can get to heaven and be remade!

I don't know how it's going to happen. A lot of days—more often than not—I get bogged down with the imaginings of everything that can go wrong. Raising three children with two parents is a huge job. Raising three broken, hurt children with only one broken, hurt parent is an astronomical, how-can-it-be-done job! But my God knows. He knows our hurts, and He can heal. That's what I pray for: healing for my sons. I don't want them to ever forget me. But I do want God to use the experience that this hurt and loss is/will be for something spectacular. I can't even imagine yet what it could be!…But God knows. And I trust Him with them…even the one who never takes his ear phones out of his ears just to make me nuts.

From This Side

May 21, 2014

I HAVE GREAT FRIENDS WHO remind me daily that I am loved.

I have a great family who takes care of me and shows love through their sacrificial giving.

I have three little boys who are my world.

And I have Jesus, who is faithful and unchanging.

"My flesh and my heart may fail, but God is the strength of my heart and my portion forever." Psalm 73:26

Many of you know that Psalm 73:26 is my life verse. These are dark, scary days when my flesh and my heart actually are failing. These are days when I desperately need something to cling to, and this is it: Jesus. He has given me everything I need. Admitted-ly, there are times I take my eyes off of Him, and that is the very second I begin to flail in overwhelming waters. I start to drown. I can not—not for one second—take my eyes off of my Light.

I have recently experienced a minor (felt major to me!) medical emergency where I could not get enough oxygen. It felt like there was not enough air in the whole world to help me breathe in a cadence that would sustain my life. So. Very. Scary. We called hospice to help, and eventually I got it under control.

It was an eye-opening experience for a lot of reasons, the main one being this: When I need medical help—REAL medical help for a REAL medical crisis—I'm not going to go to the hospital. I'm not going to call a doctor. There will be no emergency room. I'm going to call hospice. Nurse will come and she will hold my hand. Mom will tell me "It's okay," over and over again. I will feel panicked, and I am very, very afraid of that.

It's a bad feeling to live in fear. Especially when I know that the fear is unnecessary. Jesus will take care of me. But from this side, it's hard to see how that will happen. From this side, it's dark. From this side, it is terribly frightening.

I have so much. But from this side…my most hidden thoughts bubble up. He is enough. But how can it all possibly come together for good?

Longing

June 29, 2014

My world has been narrowed quite a lot in the last several weeks. Although I agreed to the terms of hospice care, I am always surprised when the next "thing" comes up and the response I get. That's not to say that I am dissatisfied with the service. In fact, I've been quite pleased with my experience. I recently had an episode in which I slept from 9:30 p.m. until 4:00 p.m. the following day. That, my friends, is a lot of sleeping! The nurse came out to make sure I was ok (I was). Since that initial day, it has happened a couple more times. On that first day when the nurse was here, I was surprised that I didn't get the reaction from her that I expected. She was very, very calm. Not negligent, not uncaring… just calm. I suppose that's how it goes in the hospice world.

I have a deep longing to be done here. If I were to be really truthful, I would tell you that I am disappointed most mornings to open my eyes and figure out that I am still here. I honestly thought I would have been taken home by now. Of course, the plans I make for myself rarely coincide with the plans that God makes for me. So, I spend a lot of my time thinking about heaven. What will it look like? Will I get to spend some one-on-one time with Jesus? Will there be lines to stand in to wait to meet the heroes of my faith: Moses, Noah, David, Peter, Peter (to name a few) like the queue at DisneyWorld?

"Eye has not seen, ear has not heard, neither has it entered into the heart of man all that God has prepared for those that love Him." 1 Corinthians 2:9

My mom wrote this verse for me and hung it on the wall where I can see it often. It is a promise I cling to with all my might. I know that there must be some reason that God is keeping me here, still alive, instead of swooping me up to be with Him. I certainly do wish I could understand it.

Instead, Monster marches on. Although my pain is well-managed, it has been necessary to take extra measures lately to ensure that that continues. I recently switched from oral meds to a pain pump. Were you to ever see me, you would notice the giant needle that is stabbed in my chest, or you might widen your eyes at the iv tubing that is attached to me, which must be carried everywhere I go. Everywhere. There's no question that the pump is the better option…I was taking as many as 30 pills each day. Still, it is cumbersome and only so much tubing will stay put in the cute Vera Bradley bag I tote around.

All that medicine is making me do weird things. Example: I had a dream where I was quite insistent that Princess Lovely come for tea. This was overheard by my mother, who is still giggling about it. Princess Lovely—ha! I also have had several instances where my hands will move while I'm sleeping. A few nights ago I tried to feed myself some imaginary yogurt with an imaginary spoon, only to wake up and find that things were just as I had left them when my eyes were closed. There was no spoon, no yogurt—just bedsheets. Bummer.

You might be wondering how my three little cowboys are holding up. Truth be told, I'm kind of wondering the same thing. It is like pulling teeth to get them to talk about it, and when we begin to scratch the surface, I get so nervous! What I do know for sure is that they are frightened and insecure—even though we are trying so hard to make it okay for them. Three individual little people = three individual needs. The hurt is huge. At times, it feels insurmountable. I have some guilt, because when this is all said and done, I get to be the lucky one. They have to stay here and learn to live without their mom. Some days seem good, and other days are very emotional and difficult. You would not waste a prayer on my three precious boys.

How about some good news? Ally's Wish is booming! Due to the generous support from so many, wishes are being granted! The Harrison family just returned from their trip to DisneyWorld. Angie was able to spend time in the parks each day with her husband the their three children, making memories that will last. Additionally, we have another mom whose wish we are already working on! She has meticulously journaled throughout her long fight with her Monster, and now she wants to have her journals bound into a book. That will be the next project for the team. It thrills me to no end that this foundation exists to make wishes come true for hurting families! As always, you can support us financially and make a difference to other people. Simply go to www.allyswish.org and click on the "donate" button. Thank you!

Please pray. Please pray that the days, however many there are left, would pass quickly—but not TOO quickly. Please pray that I would have discernment in making decisions and that the hearts of those who love me would be prepared. I am fully, 100%, no-questions-asked ready to go home. I'm thankful—-SO thankful—that this space is only temporary. You can have all this world, but give me Jesus.

Dwelling Place

Saturday, July 12, 2014

On Friday, July 11, at 11 p.m., our daughter Allyson Hendrickson went to be with Jesus. She is at home with the Lord now. The truth is that through all parts of her life—the joys and sorrows, the uncertainties and hope, the laughter and tears—He has been her constant. The Lord was her Dwelling Place on earth and this continues to be true in Heaven.

We do not consider that Allyson lost her battle with cancer. Instead, her Lord, the King of Kings, defeated the Monster for His precious daughter Allyson. She is victorious.

In honor of Allyson's bright spirit, you are invited to wear bright clothes or accessories and join us for her memorial service on Tuesday, July 15, at 2:00 p.m. at First Baptist Church Lewisville. We look forward to it with thankful hearts.

> Lord, You have been our dwelling place through all generations. Before the mountains were born or You gave birth to the earth and the world, even from everlasting to everlasting You are God. (Psalm 90:1–2)

Allyson Hendrickson

Dear Cole, Cade, and Austin,

I am sure that you have hundreds of thoughts and questions swirling around in your minds, and that you probably feel scared and sad. Maybe I can help in a tiny way by using this letter to remind you of things that are true:

Each of you is so very, very loved. Do you want to know the one thing that made me sadder and angrier than anything else about the cancer? It was that it made me feel like I could not be a very good mother for my three cowboys. I hope you will forgive the time I had to spend away from you, going to doctor visits or resting in bed at home, and instead just remember how much I loved you. We had some great times—remember how we used to drive around with all the windows rolled down and sing? "Sweet Caroline" and "My Little Buttercup" never sounded so good! I hope you will carry those memories close to your hearts.

God made you and He loves you even more than I could. You've all heard the stories of the days you were born a zillion times (sharing those stories never got old to me)! It still stops me in my tracks to consider that the God of the universe carefully crafted you, and then He hand-picked ME to be your mom. God knew that the cancer would come. God was not surprised that you would have to sit in this church today for this reason. He made us to go together! And our God does not make mistakes, sweet boys. Our family has suffered a lot, but God knows. And He cares. And because of His great love for you, you can run to Him whenever you feel scared or sad or overwhelmed. I want you to ask Jesus for help. It's what I've done for a long, long time, and He has never failed me once.

God is good. You probably don't feel like God has done you much of a favor today, do you? What kind of a God takes away a mom from her children? You know what? I don't know. All I am certain of—100% certain—is that God is good. God will give Daddy everything he needs to take care of you. God will give each of you the tools you need to grow up to be strong, amazing men. He is good, and you can take refuge in knowing that.

I am in heaven. One of the best things about heaven is that there is no more sickness—that means that there is no more cancer! In heaven, I get to be well. I'm not exactly sure what it will be like, but there is no doubt that it is beautiful and filled with good things. In heaven I won't have to be sick or sad anymore. We will see each other again there someday! Anytime you feel afraid or unsure of yourself, you can remember that you never have to be alone. You are part of me, and I am a part of you.

One day you will get to be here with me, too. That will be the best day ever! I am so proud of each one of you, and remember: I love you with my whole heart.

Love,
Mom